Gingival Enlargement

Pallavi Sharma, Dwiti Thanawala,
Alankrita Chaudhary, Himani Sharma

Contents

To update the Table of Contents, please right-click the field and choose 'Update Field' and 'Update Entire Table.' When you update the Contents field, the fonts would automatically change to the default 'Calibri' setting given by Word. You can manually select the text and change the font to 'Gandhi serif.' Please delete these instructions once you update the Table of Contents. For more details, please go through the Reference Guide.

1. Introduction

Gingival diseases are a range of diverse and complex pathological entities, confined to the gingiva, caused by numerous etiologic factors.[1] There are several characteristics common to all gingival diseases like clinical signs and symptoms of inflammation, the presence of bacterial plaque to initiate and/or aggravate the severity of the disease and also reversibility of the disease after the etiologic factor is eliminated.[1] Changes in the gingival characteristics like colour, contour, consistency, size, surface texture, shape and position aids the clinician in determining the health or disease state of the gingiva. An alteration in size is a common characteristic of gingival diseases.

An increase in the size of the gingiva is known as gingival enlargement or gingival overgrowth and it is accurately a clinical depiction of the condition[2]

Gingival enlargement can have several etiologies, such as local factors causing inflammation, systemic diseases, drugs, hereditary etc. At the 1999 International Workshop for the Classification of Periodontal Diseases organized by the American Academy of Periodontology, the various enlargements were categorized as plaque-induced gingival diseases modified by systemic diseases, medications and malnutrition and non-plaque-induced gingival diseases of genetic origin.[3] The progression and clinical characteristics of these diseases could be further influenced by genetic factors that may modify the disease susceptibility.

Gingival enlargement produces clinical symptoms including pain and tenderness, bleeding on probing or spontaneously, occlusal complications, atypical tooth movement, augmentation of development of caries and periodontal diseases, along with speech disturbances and aesthetic problems. These not only compromise the function but also the patient's quality of life.

Hence, resolution of the enlargement is a major concern of the patient as well as the clinician. Treatment of gingival enlargement is essential to achieve gingival stability, thus ensuring adequate plaque control, an improvement in function as well as esthetics. There are several techniques which help in the elimination of the enlarged gingival tissues. It can be accomplished by non-surgical methods, concomitant use of antiseptic mouthwashes and maintenance of good oral hygiene.

However, in certain cases, surgical intervention is recommended.[4]

This book highlights the etiopathogenesis and clinical features correlated with the several types of gingival enlargement, in addition to its multi-disciplinary management and prevention.

2. Classification

The classification of gingival enlargement provides a structure to systematically and scientifically study the etiopathogenesis as well as management of the disease in an organized manner.

Gingival enlargements can be classified in the following ways.[2]

I.   Based on the criteria of location and distribution of gingival enlargement

1)   Localized: Limited to the gingiva adjacent to a single tooth or a group of teeth.

2)   Generalized: Involving the gingiva throughout the mouth.

3)   Marginal: Confined to the marginal gingiva.

4)   Papillary: Confined to the interdental papilla.

5)   Diffuse: Involving the marginal gingiva, attached gingiva and the interdental papillae.

6)   Discrete: An isolated sessile or pedunculated tumor-like enlargement.

II. Based on etiologic factors and pathologic changes

1. Inflammatory Enlargement

a) Chronic

b) Acute

2. Drug-induced enlargement

3. Enlargement associated with systemic diseases or conditions

a) Conditioned enlargement

* Pregnancy

* Puberty

* Vitamin C deficiency

* Plasma cell gingivitis

* Nonspecific conditioned enlargement (Pyogenic granuloma)

b) Systemic diseases causing gingival enlargement

* Leukemia

- Granulomatous diseases (Wegeners graulomatosis, Sarcoidosis)

4. Neoplastic enlargement (Gingival tumours)

a) Benign tumours

b) Malignant tumours

5. False enlargement

3. Inflammatory Enlargement

Gingival enlargement may result from acute or chronic inflammatory changes. Additionally, inflammatory changes frequently are a secondary complication to other kinds of gingival enlargement leading to combined enlargement and hence the understanding of the dual etiology is essential to plan the treatment accordingly.[2]

Chronic Inflammatory Enlargement

When edema, inflammatory cell infiltration and vascular engorgement dominate, gingival enlargement is referred to as inflammatory gingival enlargement. When the enlarged gingivae consist essentially of dense fibrous tissue, the condition is referred to as fibrotic gingival enlargement. The term "chronic hyperplastic gingivitis" was frequently used for both processes.[5]

Etiology

Prolonged exposure to dental plaque is the predominant causative factor of chronic inflammatory gingival enlargement. Numerous factors encourage accumulation as well the retention of plaque like poor oral hygiene (Fig. 1), anatomic abnormalities, orthodontic appliances (Fig. 2), improper restorations etc. [2]

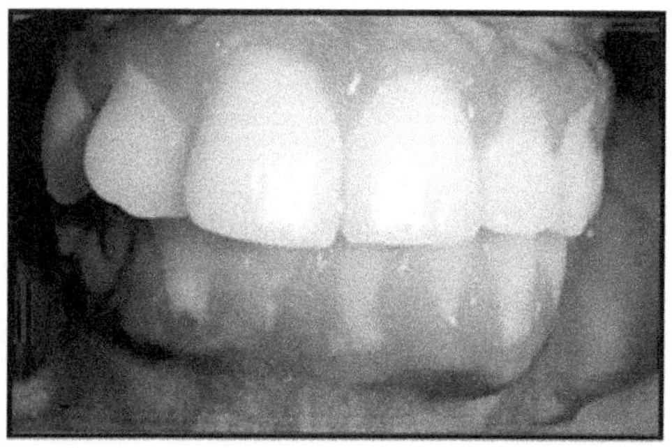

Fig 1. Chronic inflammatory enlargement

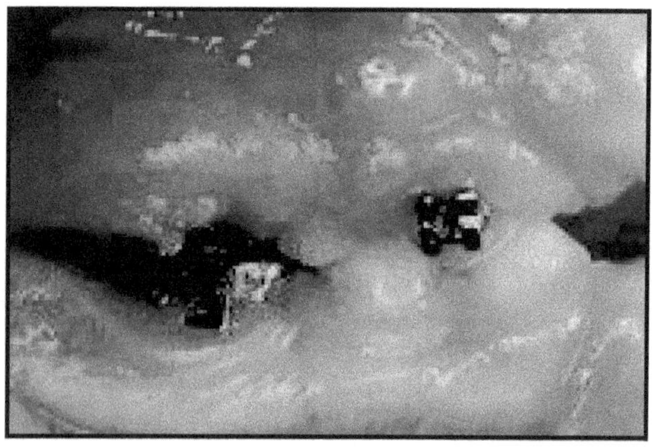

Fig 2. Enlargement due to orthodontic appliances.

Clinical Features

1.   Starts at a region of inadequate oral hygiene, food impaction or other cause of local irritation.

2.   It originates as a slight ballooning of the interdental papilla and/or the marginal gingiva.

3.   In the initial stages, may result in a life preserver-shaped inflammation all around the concerned teeth.

4.   The involved tissues are smooth, edematous, glossy and bleed spontaneously or on probing.

5.   Sometimes, it occurs as a distinct pedunculated/sessile mass akin to a tumor.

6.   The enlargement can be generalized or localized and progresses gradually and painlessly if not complicated by trauma or acute infection2

7.   The pseudo pockets formed by gingival enlargement make the oral hygiene maintenance difficult.

8.   A fetid odor may be caused due to decomposition of food debris and accumulation of bacteria in these inaccessible areas.

9.   Painful ulceration occasionally occurs in the fold between the gingiva and the inflammatory mass.

10. Loss of interdental bone and tooth migration occur in long-standing cases of inflammatory enlargement.

Histologic Features

Chronic inflammatory gingival enlargements exhibit both proliferative and exudative features of chronic inflammation. The predominance of inflammatory cells and fluid with new capillary formation, vascular engorgement, and associated degenerative changes are associated with clinically bluish-red, soft, and friable lesions with a smooth surface that bleeds easily. Relatively firm and resilient lesions have a greater fibrotic component with a large quantity of fibroblasts and collagen fibers (Fig 3). [5]

Pallavi Sharma, Dwiti Thanawala,
Alankrita Chaudhary, Himani Sharma

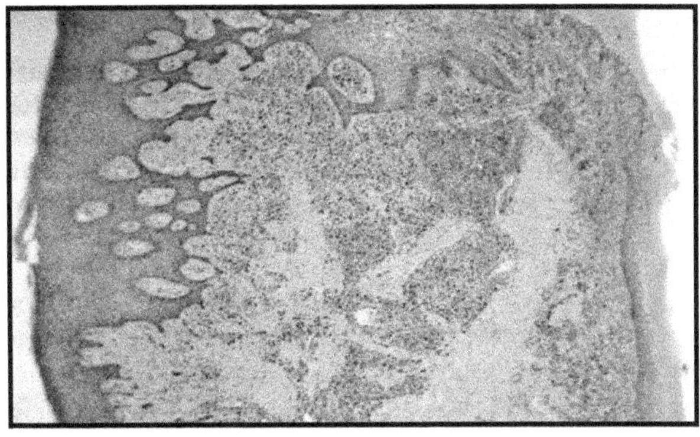

Fig 3. Histological section of chronicinflammatory gingival enlargement

Diagnosis

The diagnosis of inflammatory gingival enlargement generally presents no complication. The typical clinical feature of inflammatory gingival enlargement permits differentiation from fibrotic gingival enlargement.

Treatment

Treatment of inflammatory gingival enlargement comprises of the establishment of good oral hygiene, rectification of all local predisposing factors and eradication of any established systemic predisposing causes.

Patients with severe gingival enlargement may require surgical excision of the affected tissue followed by contouring of the remaining tissue.

Gingival Changes Associated with Mouth Breathing

Gingivitis and gingival enlargement are frequently found in mouth breathers. The gingiva appears reddish and edematous with a diffuse surface shininess. The most involved area is the maxillary anterior region. Sometimes the altered gingiva may be demarcated from the unexposed adjacent gingiva. The harmful effect is ascribed to irritation resulting from dehydration of the dehydration. The precise method in which mouth breathing affects gingival changes is not clear (Fig 4).[2]

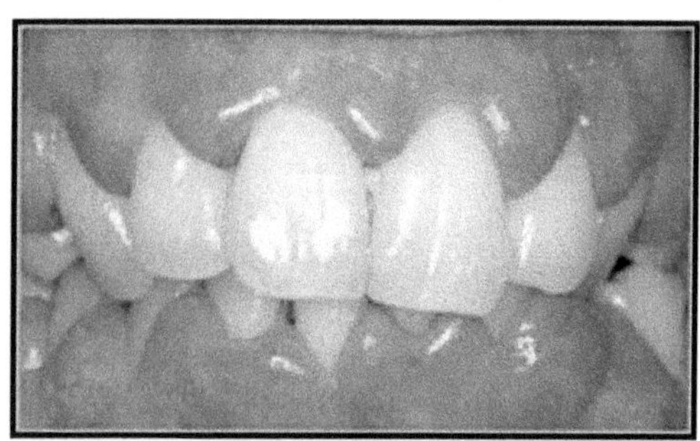

Fig 4. Enlargement associated with mouth breathing

Pallavi Sharma, Dwiti Thanawala,
Alankrita Chaudhary, Himani Sharma

Acute Inflammatory Enlargement

Acute inflammatory gingival enlargement is seen in the form of an abscess which contains purulent inflammation in the periodontal tissues.

Abscesses are one of the main causes for patients to seek out urgent care. Frequently seen in untreated periodontitis patients, it may also arise in patients receiving maintenance treatment.[6] This condition has diagnostic, prognostic, and therapeutic implications in everyday periodontal practice.[7]

Classification

Different classifications have been proposed for periodontal abscesses:

I.   Chronic

        Acute

II.   Single

        Multiple

III.   Gingival abscesses (in previously healthy sites and caused by impaction of foreign bodies)

Periodontal abscesses (either acute or chronic, in relation to a periodontal pocket)

Pericoronal abscesses (at incompletely erupted teeth). [6]

Gingival Abscess

It is a confined, painful, swiftly growing lesion involving the interdental papilla or marginal gingiva or rarely in a formerly disease-free area. Usually, it is an acute inflammatory reaction to foreign elements pushed in the gingiva and appears as an erythematous swelling with a shining smooth surface. Within 24-48 hours, the lesion frequently turns fluctuant and pointed with an orifice from which purulent exudate can be expressed.6 If allowed to progress, the lesion usually ruptures spontaneously. The adjacent teeth are frequently sensitive to percussion (Fig 5).[2]

Pallavi Sharma, Dwiti Thanawala,
Alankrita Chaudhary, Himani Sharma

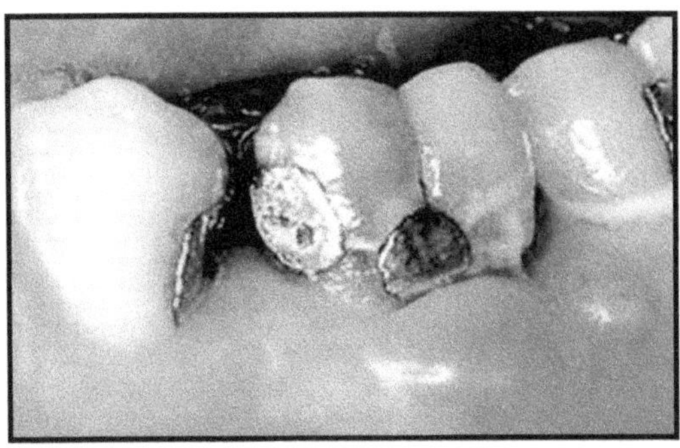

Fig 5. Gingival abscess in relation to 36 region

Histopathology

It consists of a purulent focal point in the connective tissue encircled by diffuse infiltration of PMNs, vascular engorgement and edematous tissue. The surface epithelium has variable levels of intracellular and extracellular edema, invasion by white blood cells, and occasionally ulceration.[2]

Periodontal Abscess

Definition

The periodontal abscess has been defined as a lesion with an expressed periodontal breakdown, occurring during a limited period of time, and with easily detectable clinical symptoms, with a localised accumulation of pus, located within the gingival wall of the periodontal pocket.[8]

Classification

Depending on the origin, there are two types of periodontal abscesses[9]:

1. Periodontitis-related abscess

In patients with periodontitis, a periodontal abscess denotes a specific period of active periodontal tissue breakdown. It occurs due to the expansion of the infection into intact periodontal tissues. This abscess formation occurs usually due to the marginal closure of a deep periodontal pocket, existence of deep, tortuous pockets that lack proper drainage. Once the acute inflammatory process starts, there is a local accumulation of neutrophils, tissue breakdown and pus formation. The retention of pus in the pocket further compromises the drainage and the lesion rapidly progresses into deeper parts of the periodontium. There are different mechanisms behind the formation of a periodontitis-related abscess

A.   Acute exacerbation of a chronic lesion

Such abscesses may develop in a deep periodontal pocket without any apparent external affect and may occur in an untreated periodontitis patient

B.   Post-therapy periodontal abscesses

There are distinct reasons why an abscess may occur during active therapy.

- Post-antibiotic periodontal abscess

If the cases of advanced periodontitis are treated with systemic antibiotics without subgingival debridement it can lead to abscess formation.[6,10] In such patients, the microbiota in the subgingival biofilm may be protected from the antibiotic, a super-infection may result, and massive inflammation occurs.

- Post-scaling periodontal abscess

Post-scaling periodontal abscess usually occurs immediately after a routine professional prophylaxis or scaling due to the obstruction of the entrance of the pocket by small pieces of residual calculus once the gingival edema has disappeared.

This kind of abscess can also result from embedding of small fragments of calculus into the deep, formerly uninflamed parts of the periodontal tissues.[11] In such instances the shrinking of gingival wall leads to occlusion of the pocket orifice, and the abscess happens in the sealed-off portion of the pocket.[6]

- Post-surgery periodontal abscess

When an abscess immediately forms after periodontal surgery, it is frequently the consequence of an inadequate removal of subgingival calculus or existence of foreign substances in the periodontal tissues, such as regenerative devices, sutures, or periodontal pack.[12]

- As a recurrent infection during supportive periodontal treatment.

2. Non-periodontitis-related abscess

This type of abscess may also form in relation to a periodontal pocket; however, the acute inflammation can always be attributed to external local factor that explains the acute inflammation. Such factors include

A. Impaction of foreign substance in periodontal pocket or gingival sulcus

It might be associated with oral hygiene practices (e.g. toothpicks, toothbrush, etc.), food particles, orthodontic devices etc. When the periodontal abscesses are caused by foreign bodies, related to oral hygiene aids, have been named ''oral hygiene abscesses''.[13]

B.   Root morphology alterations

In this instance local anatomical factors, such as an invaginated root or fissured root, an external root resorption, root tears or iatrogenic endodontic perforations, may be the cause of the abscess formation.

Pathogenesis and Histopathology[9]

It is recognized that a periodontal abscess is established by trauma or occlusion to the periodontal pocket orifice, causing the infection to extend to the soft tissues of the pocket wall. An inflammatory infiltrate is formed leading to the destruction of the connective tissues followed by the encapsulation of the bacterial accumulation and eventually formation of purulent exudate (Fig 6). The inflammatory cells and extracellular enzymes are primarily responsible for the tissue destruction. The initiation of the pocket formation is due to the entry of bacteria into the soft tissue pocket wall and the bacterial virulence decreased tissue resistance determines the course of the infection.

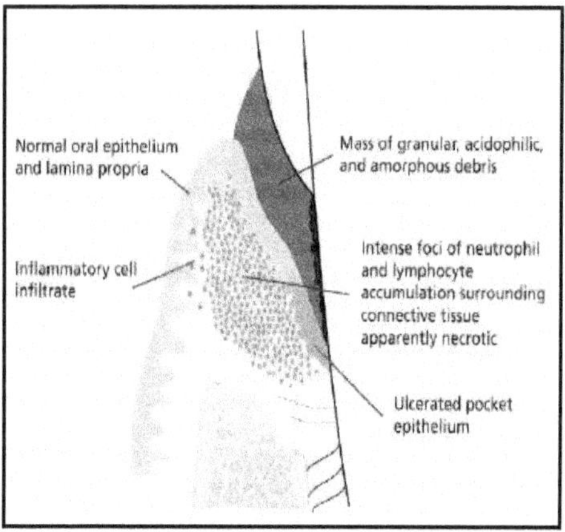

Fig 6. Schematic drawing showing the histopathology of a periodontal abscess

A periodontal abscess includes bacteria and bacterial products, tissue breakdown products, serum, and inflammatory cells. Histologically, PMNs are found in the central part of the abscess and near soft tissue debris. Subsequently, a pyogenic membrane is formed consisting of neutrophils and macrophages. The local pH, the growing of bacteria inside the foci and their virulence determines the rate of tissue destruction.[8]

Microbiology

Purulent oral infections are polymicrobial and produced by endogenous microorganisms. Sixty percent of cultured bacteria were strict anaerobes, most frequently gram-negative anaerobic rods, and gram-positive facultative cocci. In general, gram-negatives dominated over gram-positives and rods over cocci14. Higher proportions of spirochetes and low proportions of cocci and motile rods are found. Culture studies have shown Fusobacterium spp (75%), P. intermedia/ nigrescens (60%) and P. gingivalis (51.7%) were the maximum prevalent microorganisms.15 However, other microorganisms like Campylobacter rectus (80%), Aggregatibacter actinomycetemcomitans (25%), and Prevotella melaninogenica (22%) have likewise been reported.[14] Bacterial species which produce proteinases, such as P. intermedia, are essential, because they improve the accessibility of nutrients, and thereby, enhance the number of bacteria inside the abscess.

Clinical Features

1.   An ovoid elevation of gingiva along the lateral part of the tooth root. However, abscesses which are deep in the periodontium may be less obvious (Fig 7).

2.   Mandibular anterior teeth are affected the most, followed by maxillary anterior teeth and mandibular molars (Fig 8).[15]

3.   Symptoms may vary from little discomfort to severe pain, tenderness of the gingiva, swelling, tooth elevation, tooth mobility, sensitivity to palpation.[16]

4.   Bleeding on probing may be seen commonly along with suppuration, either spontaneous or following pressure on the abscess, come together with deep pocket formation.[16]

5.   Halitosis has also been reported.

6.   Systemic involvement has been stated in severe cases including malaise, fever, leukocytosis, and regional lymphadenopathy.[16]

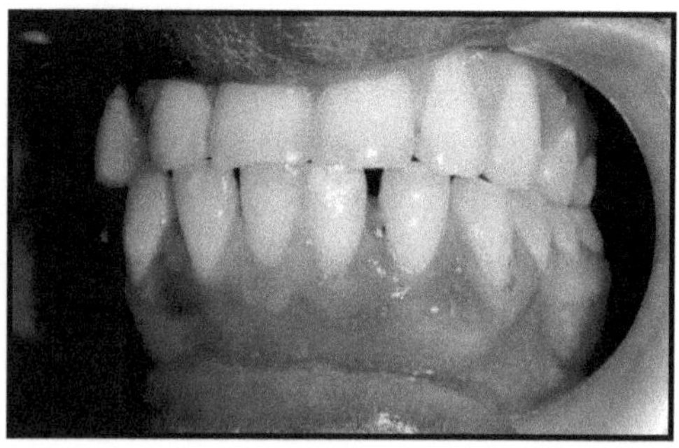

Fig 7. Periodontal abscess in relation to 32, 33.

Pallavi Sharma, Dwiti Thanawala,
Alankrita Chaudhary, Himani Sharma

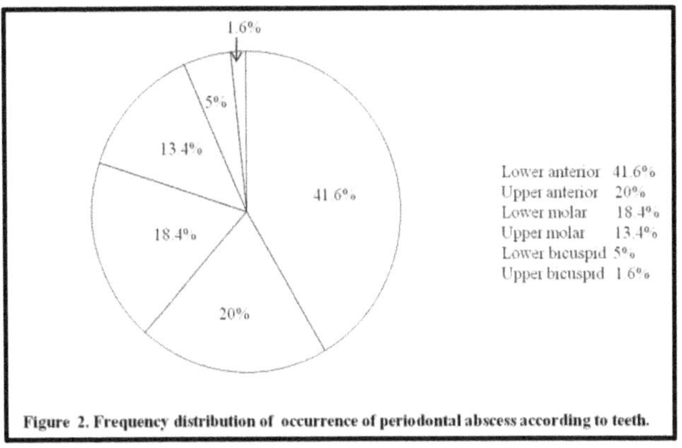

Figure 2. Frequency distribution of occurrence of periodontal abscess according to teeth.

Fig 8. Frequency distribution of periodontal abscess according to teeth

Radiographic Examination

The radiographic examination may show a normal appearance or some amount of bone loss, varying from only widening of the periodontal space to a critical bone loss (Fig 9).

Van Winkelhoff et al. (1985) instituted a diagnostic criterion for the defining of a periodontal abscess:

1.   Association with pockets greater than or equal to 6 mm

2.   Bleeding on probing

3.   Radiographic alveolar bone loss and absence of a periapical lesion

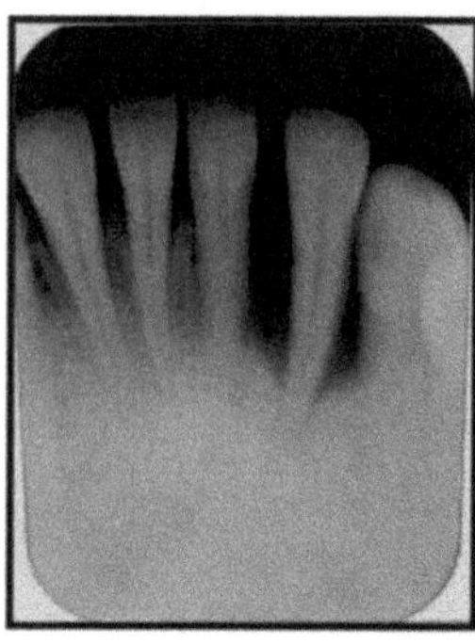

Fig 9. Radiograph of periodontal abscess in relation to 32, 33.

Laboratory Investigations

Dark-field microscopic examination can help exclude an endodontic origin, due to the greater proportion of spirochetes in periodontal abscesses.

Liu et al. (1996) suggested the use of positron emission tomography and a flurine-18-fluoromisonidazole marker for recognition of periodontal abscesses and other anaerobic infections in the oral cavity. The technique was effective in recognition of 100% of periodontal abscesses.[7]

Laboratory data from blood and urine of patients immediately after a periodontal abscess reported that in 30% of the patients there were an elevated number of leukocytes. The absolute number of blood neutrophils and monocytes was also enhanced in 20-40% of the patients. [7]

Diagnosis

Diagnosis of a periodontal abscess is established with the help of total evaluation and interpretation of the patient's chief complaint and the clinical and radiological signs observed during the oral examination. Further information is acquired through a meticulous dental and medical history.

Differential Diagnosis [9]

1.   Acute infections such as lateral periapical cysts, periapical abscesses, endo-periodontal abscesses, vertical root fractures and may have a similar appearance and symptoms as a periodontal abscess, although with a clearly different etiology. Signs such as absence of pulp vitality, the presence of a sinus tract, existence of deep carious lesions, and radiographic findings help in differentiating between abscesses of distinct etiologies.

2.   Other lesions may appear with a similar appearance to a periodontal abscess. Three cases of

osteomyelitis in periodontitis patients were initially diagnosed as periodontal abscess. Parrish et al. (1989)

3.   Various tumors may have the appearance of a periodontal abscess. Example: metastatic carcinoma from pancreatic origin, gingival squamous cell carcinoma, an eosinophilic granuloma.

Pericoronal Abscess

It is a localized accumulation of pus within the overlying gingival flap surrounding the crown of an incompletely erupted tooth, usually occurring in the third molar area. The gingival flap looks swollen and red (Fig 10,11).

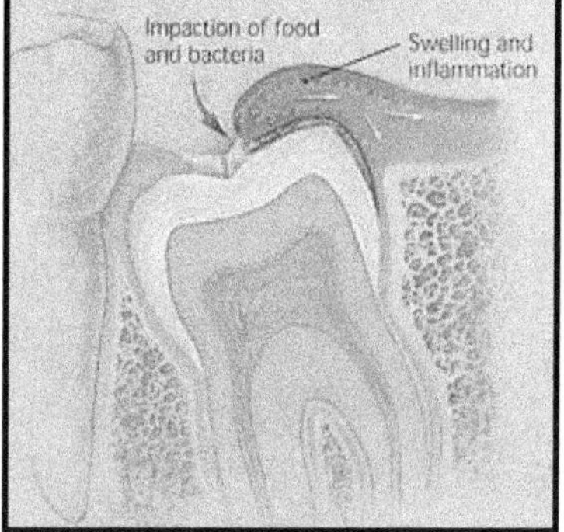

Fig 10. Schematic diagram showing inflamed coronal flap

Pallavi Sharma, Dwiti Thanawala,
Alankrita Chaudhary, Himani Sharma

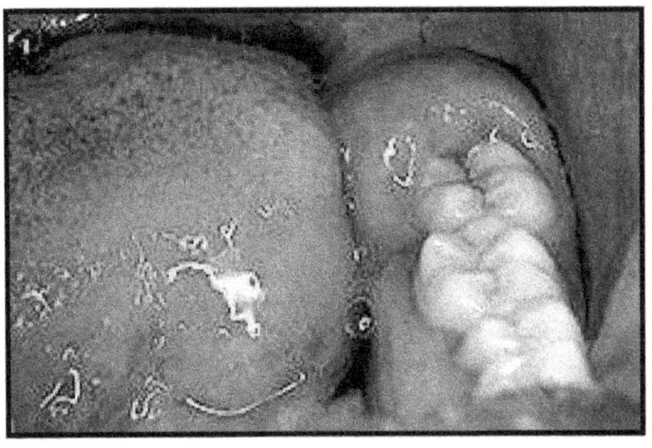

Fig 11. Pericoronal abscess in relation to 37 region

The infection may spread medially to the base of the tongue, posteriorly to the oro-pharyngeal area and involve the regional lymph nodes. Patients generally have a prior history of pericoronitis and may have trouble swallowing. A few patients may exhibit fever, malaise, or leukocytosis. An increase in the proportions of gram-negative anaerobic pathogens has been associated with the severity of pericoronitis and development of abscess formation.[6]

4. Drug Induced Gingival Enlargement

Drug induced gingival overgrowth occurs as a side effect of drug used mainly for non-dental treatment for which the gingival tissue is not the intended target organ. It is a well-known consequence of the administration of some anticonvulsants, immunosuppressants, and calcium channel blockers.[2]

Anticonvulsant drugs, calcium channel blockers and immunosuppressants are associated with disproportionate, disfiguring and functionally compromising overgrowth of gingival tissues.[17] Clinically and histologically, the gingival overgrowth due to these drugs are similar. Although there are many theories about the pathogenesis of this condition, a common unifying link between these drugs has not been established. Three significant factors which are important in the expression of these gingival changes can be considered: drug variables, plaque-induced inflammatory changes in the gingival tissues and genetic factors, the latter determining the heterogeneity of the gingival fibroblasts. Some drugs induce a direct effect on a subgroup of fibroblasts, named responders that are apparently genetically determined to be sensitive to the drug-causing gingival overgrowth.[18]

The target cell is the gingival fibroblast, as all lesions are characterized by an increase in the connective tissue component. Gingival inflammation also appears to be an important predisposing factor to this unwanted effect. This suggests that the lesion is a consequence of the interaction between gingival fibroblasts, the cellular and biochemical mediators of inflammation and the drug or its metabolites.[19]

The specific mechanism by which drug-induced gingival enlargement occurs is yet not clear, although several hypotheses have been suggested like like interaction of Phenytoin with subtype of susceptible fibroblasts, effect of cyclosporin on the metabolism of the fibroblasts and nifedipine reduces the metabolism of fibroblasts and enhances its action on fibroblasts. Various factors like age, genetic predisposition, pharmacokinetic variables, drug-induced alterations in gingival connective tissue homeostasis, drug-induced action on growth factors, etc. may affect the relationship between the various implicated drugs and components of the gingival tissues. [18]

Anticonvulsants

Drugs which are prophylactically administered to prevent the occurrence of convulsions are called anticonvulsants.

Classification [20]

Hydantoin Derivatives	Phenytoin, Ethotoin, Mephenytoin
Barbiturates	Phenobarbitone
Deoxybarbiturates	Primidone
Iminostilbenes	Carbamazepine
Succinimide	Ethosuximide
Aliphatic Carboxylic Acid	Sodium valproate
Benzodiazepine	Clonazepam, Diazepam, Clobazam
Phenyltriazine	Lamotrigine
Cyclic GABA Analogue	Gabapentin
Newer Drugs	Vigabatrin, Topiramate, Tiagabine, Levetiracetam

Drugs that are known to induce gingival overgrowth include phenytoin, ethotoin, mephenytoin, ethosuximide, methsuximide, sodium valproate, phenobarbitone and vigabatrin.[2]

Phenytoin

In 1908 Phenytoin was introduced as a barbiturate analogue, but abandoned due to poor sedative property.[20] Meritt and Putnam, introduced it clinically in 1938 to control seizure disorders in epileptic patients and in a short span of its clinical use, reports linking phenytoin to gingival overgrowth appeared in the literature.[17] The first reported case of phenytoin -induced gingival overgrowth was reported in 1939 by Kimball[21] and Faurbye in the same year. In 1959 it was suggested by Strean and Leoni that phenytoin alkalinity might be the basis of gingival overgrowth. Brandon in 1948 hypothesized that phenytoin has a direct action on the gingival tissues. In 1975, Angelopoulos claimed that phenytoin-induced degranulation of mast cells resulted in the generation of a substance that increased collagen formation. Larmas, in 1976, proposed that phenytoin had a proliferating effect mainly on the basal cell layer of the oral epithelium leading to increase in the epithelium-connective tissue interface area, confirmed by Hassel et al. The oral epithelium may have an inducing effect on the underlying fibroblasts, in which specifically alkaline phosphatase may be involved. It was speculated by Vogel in 1977 that end-organ folic acid deficiency resulted in phenytoin induced gingival enlargement, which made the gingival tissues susceptible to inflammation by causing degenerative changes in the gingival sulcular epithelium, the main physical barrier against local irritants.[18]

Mechanism of Action[20]

On the neuronal membrane phenytoin is found to have a stabilizing influence. It prevents repetitive detonation of normal brain cells during depolarization shift that happens in epileptic patients and comprises of a synchronous and large depolarization over which action potentials are superimposed. To achieve this the inactivated state of voltage sensitive neuronal Na+ channels are prolonged, and it governs the refractory period of the neuron, resulting in inhibition of high frequency discharges with mild effect on normal low frequency discharges. This effect can be observed at therapeutic doses whereas at higher concentrations effects like reduction in Ca++ influx during depolarization, glutamate inhibition and facilitation of GABA responses can be shown and intracellular accumulation of sodium during repetitive firing is also prevented. So, phenytoin selectively depresses the motor cortex of the central nervous system and is believed to facilitate this action by stabilizing neuronal discharge and restraining the progression of neuronal excitation by blocking or interfering with calcium influx across cell membranes.[17]

Pharmacokinetics

Phenytoin is said to be a weak acid with poor solubility and absorbed slowly from the gastrointestinal tract on oral administration. The drug is metabolized in the liver by microsomal enzymes i.e. members of the cytochrome P450 enzyme family, CYP2CP and is bound to plasma proteins (90%). 5-(parahydroxy drug phenyl)-5-phenylhydantoin (5-p-HPPH) is the major metabolite of Phenytoin. About 10% of them remain free and active. The side effects are usually due to excess, available free drug. Some other undesirable effects of phenytoin apart from gingival overgrowth include cardiac arrhythmias, depression of the central nervous system, drowsiness, hirsutism and osteomalacia.

Phenytoin-Induced Gingival Enlargement

The gingival enlargement prevalence rate in patients on phenytoin therapy is suggested to be fifty percent[4]

Clinical Features (Fig .1)

1. More common in young patients.

2. The facial gingiva of the anterior sextants is found to be involved more frequently and usually results in esthetic disFig.ment.[17]

3. Initial enlargement of the interdental papilla is a common characteristic whereas increased thickening of the marginal tissue is not very common.

4. Affected tissue presents a granular or pebbly surface appearance, with the distended papillae extending facially and or lingually, obscuring the tissue adjacent to it and tooth surfaces. Clinical presence of pseudo clefts is seen as the outcome of enlarged papillae.[17]

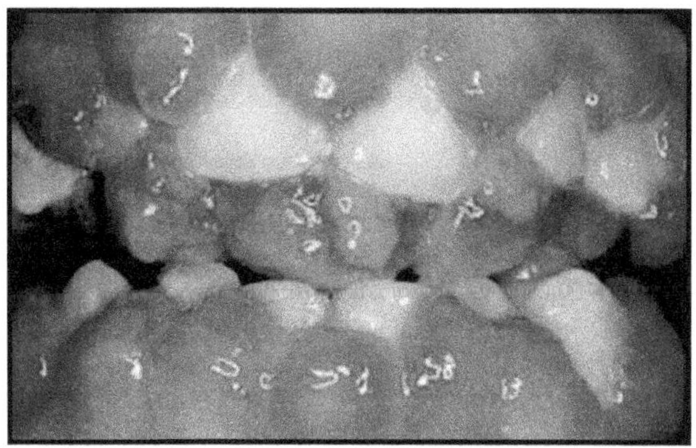

Fig 1. Phenytoin induced gingival enlargement

5.   Florid tissue overgrowth usually reduces as it comes near the mucogingival junction, coronal development may partially or totally obscure the crowns of the teeth.

6.   If it precedes the eruption of the primary teeth, it might result in delayed eruption.

7.   According to a case report of an edentulous patient, four dental implants were sited in an area without any tissue enlargement. After a period of eighteen months gingival overgrowth was noted around each implant abutment and corresponded to an increase in the patient's phenytoin dosage 3 months earlier.[22] This is a vital finding in the prospective dental implant patients consuming phenytoin.

8.   Gingival tissue enlargement can even result in malpositioning of teeth and might also interfere with normal masticatory function, oral hygiene and speech.

9.   It also makes plaque control tedious, resulting in secondary inflammatory process that further complicates the drug induced gingival hyperplasia.

10. Once the drug is discontinued the enlargement disappears spontaneously within a few months.

Histologic Features

1.   Numerous variations have been detected in both epithelium and connective tissue in phenytoin-induced gingival overgrowth.[19] Gingival overgrowth cultures present a thick stratified squamous epithelium with long thin rete pegs, regularly acanthotic, that outspread deep into the lamina propria (Fig 2).[17]

2.   The lamina propria has characteristic proliferation of fibroblasts and increased collagen formation along with an increase in non-collagenous proteins.

3.   Cultures of gingival fibroblasts from patients with phenytoin-induced gingival overgrowth presented augmented synthesis of glycosaminoglycans. It is however not clear whether this increase is because of increased amalgamation or reduced degradation.

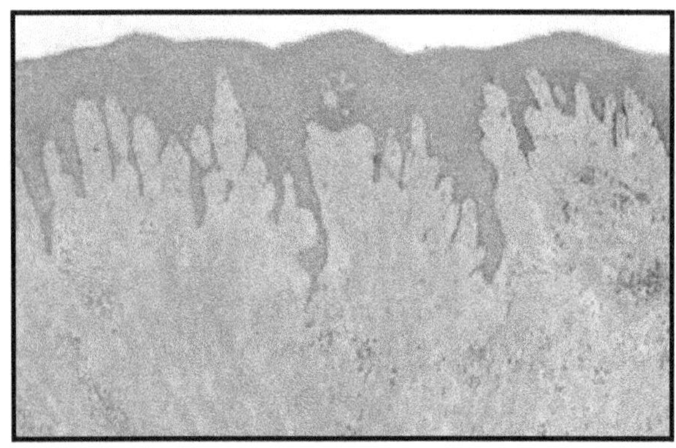

Fig 2. Histological section of cyclosporin-induced
gingival enlargement

4.　According to a study done by Haim et al 1955, collagen fibers appear thinner and shorter in comparison to those in gingiva from normal individuals.

5.　20 % of the dry weight in gingival tissues is comprised of non-collagenous proteins comprise in patients on phenytoin as compared to only 7 % in normal patients.[19]

6.　The degree of inflammation in the biopsy will determine the occurrence and range of polymorphonuclear leucocytes in the gingival epithelium.

7. Patients on extended phenytoin therapy have suggestively higher levels of hexosamine, uronic acid, and total proteins.

8. Alkaline phosphatase activity is found to be more in such tissues.[19]

Pathogenesis

Numerous mechanisms by which phenytoin might affect gingival overgrowth have been proposed.

Phenytoin and fibroblasts

The normal human gingiva holds several phenotypically different and genotypically distinct subpopulations of fibroblasts, few of which can generate huge amounts of proteins and collagen (high activity fibroblasts) and others which are capable of low protein synthesis (low activity fibroblasts). The proportion of high to low activity fibroblasts seems to be genetically determined. The high activity fibroblasts, in the existence of certain predisposing factors (eg. inflammation), become sensitive to phenytoin, with a subsequent rise in collagen making, while phenytoin or its metabolites will have no result on the low activity fibroblasts. Instead, phenytoin or its metabolites could be cytotoxic to low activity fibroblasts, thus allowing an increase in the making of high activity fibroblasts.[23]

In usual conditions, collagen produced from fibroblasts is controlled by the synchronization of transcriptional and post-translation collagen regulatory mechanisms, including intracellular degradation. Contact of gingival fibroblasts to phenytoin adds to the level of translatable collagen RNA. Excessive generation of collagen by gingival fibroblasts in phenytoin-induced gingival overgrowth contains an increased firm state level of collagen mRNA and not a reduction in collagen degradation. Such fibroblasts may be chosen during the development of overgrowth. Phenytoin could also damage degradation of collagen by reducing the enzymatic degradation with matrix metalloproteinases (MMPs), tissue inhibitors of matrix metalloproteinases and $\alpha2\beta1$ integrin-mediated endocytosis.[24]

Phenytoin and epidermal growth factor

A link has been observed between phenytoin and epidermal growth factor. Epidermal growth factor is a polypeptide in saliva that is recognized to stimulate glycosaminoglycan synthesis and stimulate influx of calcium ions into mammalian fibroblasts in vitro. It has been acknowledged as a facilitator of extracellular matrix deposition in connective tissue. Patients receiving phenytoin and are found with or without related overgrowth, epidermal growth factor receptor metabolism was downregulated in responder fibroblasts and upregulated in non-responder fibroblasts.[25]

Phenytoin and platelet-derived growth factor

It has been suggested by various authors that phenytoin increases the production of a dynamic cytokine helps in the process of connective tissue growth known as platelet-derived growth factor which can further enable gingival overgrowth.[26]

Phenytoin and folic acid

A link between phenytoin-induced gingival overgrowth and folic acid has been suggested. As an outcome of its contribution in DNA synthesis, tissues with higher turnover rates (such as epithelium) are often affected first. Folic acid deficit mainly affects the epithelium, gonads and bone marrow. Phenytoin may inhibit folic acid absorption and metabolism. The outcome may be impaired maturation of the gingival sulcular epithelium, thus making the underlying connective tissue more susceptible to inflammation. It has been noticed that systemic folic acid may be clinically helpful in deferring the onset and dropping the incidence and severity of overgrowth. It could be because of

i)   Obstruction by folic acid in the production of p-HPPH.

ii)   Competitive friction between phenytoin and folic acid which is found to be clinically important but not statistically substantial.[27]

<u>Immunosuppression</u>

Long term usage of phenytoin leads to immunosuppression and may be a contributing factor to gingival overgrowth but is not likely to be the only cause. Effect of phenytoin on immune function include lack of circulating IgA, incapability to form antibodies to different kinds of antigen challenge, decrease in the ability to manifest delayed hypersensitivity reactions and depression of lymphocyte transformation.

In the gingival tissues, secretory IgA is the first line of defense against bacterial plaque. Decrease in the IgA levels will make the tissues more prone to inflammation. Aarli et al (1976) mentioned that it is the effort of the body to deal with this inflammation via the repair processes that cause gingival enlargement.[19] Reducing both the humoral and cell mediated immune responses will result in a decrease of lymphokine production, formation of antigen-antibody complexes and complement activation. These factors together either directly or indirectly, are responsible for activating osteoclasts and hence induce bone resorption.

Phenytoin and the adrenal glands

Phenytoin therapy may lead to repression of adrenocorticotrophic hormone formation and a resultant change in pituitary-adrenal activity.[19] Depressing the adrenocortical function results in a decrease of glucocorticoid synthesis. This results in a compensatory rise in the somatotrophic hormone, a hormone that causes fibroblast proliferation.

Phenytoin also produces the sodium pump, which acts as a stimulus to fibroblasts.[19]

Phenytoin and calcium metabolism

Phenytoin acts by steadying neuronal cell membrane to the act of sodium, potassium and calcium. It also affects the passage of calcium ions across membranes by reducing membrane permeability and blocking intracellular uptake. According to the study done by Pandiella et al, fluctuations in the calcium metabolism of gingival fibroblasts may be important in the pathogenesis of the overgrowth.[19]

Thus, the accurate pathogenesis of phenytoin-induced gingival overgrowth is unclear. Several factors like direct effect of phenytoin on specific subpopulations of fibroblasts, genetic predisposition, intracellular calcium metabolism exchange, molecular mechanisms (cytokines such as epidermal growth factor, platelet-derived growth factor- P), inactivation of collagenase and inflammation induced by bacterial plaque are found to be responsible for contributing in this condition.[19,23,25,26.] The essential disorder is in the gingival fibroblast and protein synthesis. The cell is subjected to a variety of chemical messengers that are improved when the tissues are inflamed and phenytoin or its metabolites act on these chemical messengers directly or via receptors.

Other Anticonvulsants

Sodium Valproate

Valproic acid in comparison to various anticonvulsants has a broad spectrum of antiepileptic activity. Sodium valproate can be a better choice to phenytoin as it has moderately low risk for developing gingival enlargement. Number of cases of gingival overgrowth post sodium valproate are very less and these most likely signify idiosyncratic hypersensitivities.[17]

Phenobarbitone

Enlarged gingiva regularly deprived of lobulation of the interdental papillae can be seen in phenobarbitone-induced gingival overgrowth cases. Gingival Overgrowth can be more severe in the posterior regions as compared to the anterior region and can be conflicting to most other drug-induced gingival overgrowth. The histological and clinical appearance was identical to familial forms of gingival fibromatosis and, however there was no family history in these cases, it is likely that the gingival signs are part of a syndrome and the phenobarbitone therapy just occurs to be mutual to both.

Generally, these cases reply well to surgical excision and good oral hygiene appears to prevent recurrence.

Vigabatrin

Vigabatrin is comparatively a new anticonvulsant drug, which acts as a selective, unalterable inhibitor of the acid transaminase of gamma-amino butyric acid (GABA) which is the primary inhibitory neurotransmitter in the brain. Two months after initiating vigabatrin therapy a case of vigabatrin-induced gingival overgrowth was first noted and epithelial thickening with elongated rete pegs and discreetly dense foci of chronic inflammatory cells in the connective tissue was observed on histological examination. There was no response of gingival overgrowth to conservative periodontal therapy and post gingivectomy recurrence was seen. But this overgrowth was not seen in other cases and so it is presumed that this reaction was an idiosyncratic hypersensitivity.[28]

Immunosuppressants

These are drugs which are used to inhibit cellular and/or humoral immune responses and thus, have their major use in organ transplantation and autoimmune diseases.[20]

Classification

• Specific T cell inhibitor (Calcineurin inhibitors): Cyclosporin, Tacrolimus

• Cytotoxic drugs (Antiproliferative drugs): Azathioprine, Cyclophosphamide, Methotrexate, Chlorambucil

• Glucocorticoids: Prednisolone and others

• Antibodies: Muromonab CD3, Rh (D) immunoglobulin

Cyclosporin

Cyclosporin is a hydrophobic, cyclic endecapeptide derived from the metabolic products of two fungal species, Trichoderma polysporum and Cylindrocarpon lucidium. It was first isolated in Switzerland in 1970.[19] Cyclosporin, formerly known as Cyclosporin A was discovered by Jean Borel, and its first reported use was by Calne et al in renal transplantation procedures. The drug was initially produced as an antimicrobial, but investigations showed that it had an inhibitory effect on lymphocyte proliferation.[17] It suppress some humoral immunity (B lymphocytes); and to a much greater extent, cell-mediated immunity (T lymphocytes) such as allograft rejection, delayed hypersensitivity, graft-versus-host disease and autoimmune diseases. Because of its immunosuppressive action, it prolongs the survival of allogeneic transplants involving skin, heart, kidneys, liver, pancreas, bone marrow, small intestine and lungs.

Mechanism of Action [29]

The pharmacodynamics of cyclosporin mainly involve the T cell response and the role of these cells in graft rejection is shown in Fig 3

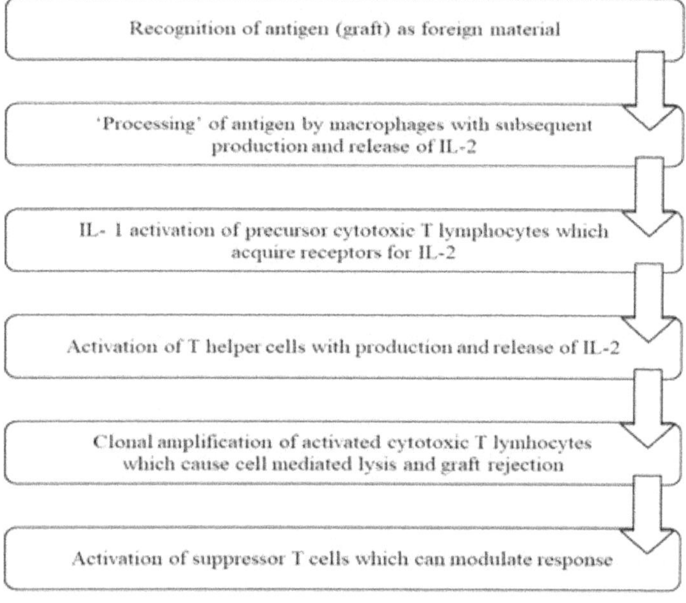

Fig 3. Mechanism of action of cyclosporin

Cyclosporin inhibits many of the above stages. Specifically, it inhibits IL-2 synthesis at concentrations between 10-20 ng/ml. Such inhibition limits clonal amplification of cytotoxic T cells. At higher concentrations (100 ng/ml), cyclosporin inhibits the ability of cytotoxic T cells to respond to IL-2. By contrast, cyclosporin has a sparing effect on suppressor T cells (Hess et al 1982).

Thus, suppressor T cells seem to be resistant to cyclosporin, whereas cytotoxic T cells and T helper cells are sensitive to the drug. These differential properties of cyclosporin on various subsets of T lymphocytes may be due to the binding properties between the drug and the cell and subsequent internalization of cyclosporin molecules into the cell structure.

Within the T cell, the drug binds to two proteins: calmodulin and cyclophilin. It has been postulated that the resistance or sensitivity of T cells to cyclosporin may be related to the proportionate intracellular concentrations of these proteins. An increase in cyclophilin will increase cyclosporin binding and thus prevent the drug from interacting with calmodulin. Conversely, low levels of cyclophilin will allow binding with calmodulin and inhibit its formation and subsequent T cell activation.

Pharmacokinetics

Cyclosporin can be given orally, intramuscularly or intravenously. After oral administration, the drug is absorbed from the gastrointestinal tract and absorption shows marked interindividual variation. It is water insoluble, and absorption depends on the presence of bile salts. Peak plasma concentrations occur 3-4 hours after dosage, and the drug has a serum half-life of approximately 17-40 hours. It is extensively metabolized in the liver and metabolism is mediated through the cytochrome P450 mono-oxygenase system. The metabolism of the drug involves N-demethylation, hydroxylation and cyclization. Some of the metabolites identified in humans are 1, 17 and 21 (Fig. 5).[19] Most of the metabolites are excreted via the bile through feces, with only 10% excreted through the kidneys. Impairment of liver or renal function may alter adequate absorption and excretion, leading to high blood levels of the drug.

The adverse side effects of cyclosporin include gingival overgrowth and multiple systemic effects. Most of these effects are dose-dependent and are frequently reversible without sequelae upon decrease or discontinuance of the drug. Nephrotoxicity is well documented and reversible, showing oliguria and weight gain related to high serum trough levels. Hepatotoxicity occurs less frequently than nephrotoxicity and is characterized by elevated serum bilirubin, transaminase and alkaline phosphatase levels, all of which are reversible via dose reduction. Hypertension is a common finding, with an incidence ranging from 38.5% to 51.2% in studies of renal transplant cases. Other less common side effects include lymphomas, Kaposi's sarcoma, squamous cell carcinoma, hyperuricemia, hyperkalemia, mild anemia, neurotoxicity, visual disturbances, depression, hypertrichosis and a predisposition to bacterial, viral and fungal infections.[17]

Cyclosporin-Induced Gingival Overgrowth

The prevalence rate of gingival overgrowth in patients on cyclosporin therapy ranges from 25-50%. The reasons for this range are many and include the nature of the disease being treated, the age of the patient, the method of assessment, the dosage and duration of cyclosporin and additional medications if any.[4,30] Studies have shown oral doses over 500 mg/day resulted in gingival enlargement, while doses below 300 mg/day did not, which implied that a threshold concentration is required for gingival enlargement.[29] The first cases of gingival overgrowth caused by cyclosporin medication in the dental literature were reported by Rateitschak-Pluss et al.[17,19,30] They studied 50 kidney transplant patients, most of whom developed gingival enlargement after 4-6 weeks of cyclosporin treatment. None demonstrated recurrence after the teeth were extracted.

Clinical Features (Fig 4)

1.   A greater risk of developing cyclosporin-induced gingival enlargement is seen in children, especially adolescents and young females. The reason could be a possible interaction between cyclosporin, sex hormones and gingival fibroblasts.

2.   Gingival overgrowth is usually seen 3 months after dosage.

3.   It normally begins at the interdental papillae and is more common in the anterior segments of the mouth and on labial surfaces of the teeth. It is not seen in edentulous patients.

4. The enlarged gingival tissues are soft, red or bluish red, extremely fragile and bleed easily upon probing.

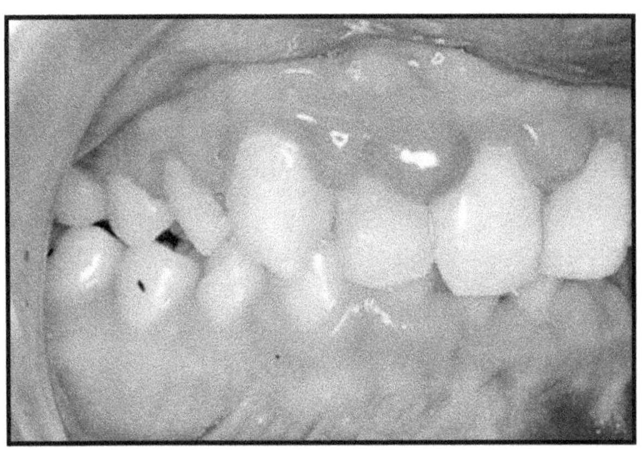

Fig 4. Cyclosporin- induced gingival enlargement

5. It is more vascularized than the phenytoin-induced enlargement[2,30]

6. Overgrowth is restricted to keratinized gingiva but could extend coronally and interfere with occlusion, mastication and speech.

7. Rostock et al. reported spontaneous repositioning of migrated teeth after removal of the enlarged tissue, resulting in visible narrowing of diastema as early as 2 months after surgery, indicating

that the toot migration could be result of cyclosporin-induced gingival overgrowth.[31]

8.   Gingival enlargement is greater in patients who are medicated with both cyclosporin and calcium channel-blocking drugs.[32,33,34,35] It has been suggested that combined therapy may increase the prevalence of the condition but not the severity and that it is a significant risk factor for progression and recurrence of the lesion after treatment.

HISTOLOGIC FEATURES (Fig 5)

1.   It consists primarily of connective tissue with an overlying multilayered, irregular, parakeratinized epithelium of variable thickness.

2.   Epithelial ridges penetrate deep into the connective tissue, creating irregularly arranged collagen fiber bundles.

3.   Acanthosis and parakeratinization of the epithelium with pseudoepitheliomatous proliferation is also noted.

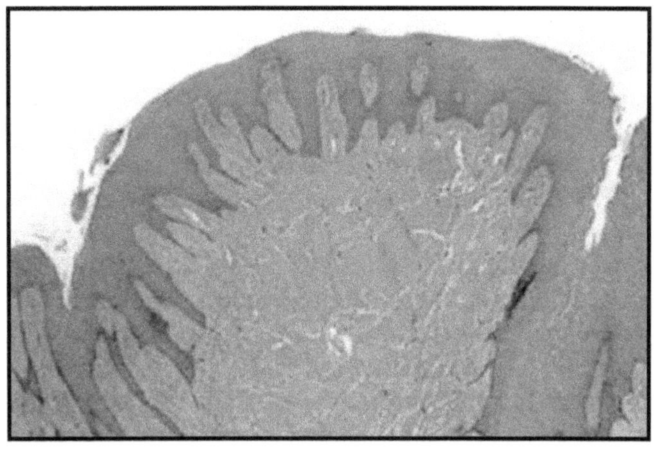

Fig 5 Histological section of cyclosporin-induced gingival enlargement

4.   Focal areas of myxomatous change have been seen more often in the immediate subepithelial tissue than in deeper areas.[17,19]

5.   The connective tissue is highly vascularized, and focal accumulations of infiltrating inflammatory cells have been seen. The predominant cell type in the inflammatory infiltrate is the plasma cell, with lymphocytes seen to a lesser degree. The mononuclear cell infiltrate has demonstrated the presence of T lymphocytes and monocytes adjacent to the junctional epithelium, with virtually no B lymphocytes.[17,19]

6.   No increase in numerical density of fibroblasts, which has led to the impression that cyclosporin-induced gingival enlargement, is a result of an accumulation of non-collagenous material and a thickening of the epithelium.[17]

7.   Electron microscopic examination of gingival fibroblasts revealed ultrastructural characteristics of active protein synthesis and secretion, with reduced cytotoxic or degenerative changes.

Pathogenesis

The pathogenesis of cyclosporin-gingival overgrowth is truly multifactorial and remains uncertain despite numerous investigative studies. Three significant factors appear to be important to the expression of gingival overgrowth: drug   variables,   plaque-induced inflammatory changes in the gingiva and genetic factors.[21]

Since fewer than 50% of patients taking cyclosporin develop gingival enlargement, the terms "responders" and "nonresponders" have been used to identify these individual   differences   and   perhaps   a   genetic predisposition.

Wysocki et al. (1983) suggested that gingival overgrowth was related to sensitivity of individuals to the drug or its metabolites. Cyclosporin and its major metabolite OL-17 could react with a phenotypically distinct subpopulation of gingival fibroblasts, causing an increase in protein synthesis and rate of cell proliferation. Coley et al. (1986) demonstrated that the effects of cyclosporin on normal human fibroblast proliferation varied among individual cell strains, where strains were shown to increase, decrease, or remain unchanged.[17]

There are marked differences among fibroblast strains for collagenase and tissue inhibitor of metalloproteinase production when exposed to cyclosporin, which may explain in part the variable gingival response in patients taking this drug. Collagen production from gingival fibroblasts is controlled by synthesis and release of metalloproteinases and tissue inhibitor of metalloproteinases. In vitro studies have shown that cyclosporin causes a significant increase in collagen synthesis, but not DNA synthesis, with a specific rise in the level of type I procollagen.[17]

Another factor that may relate to the expression of drug-induced gingival overgrowth is human lymphocyte antigen (HLA). It was noted that patients who expressed HLA-DR1 appeared to have a protective role against gingival overgrowth from cyclosporin, whereas those expressing HLA-DR2 showed an increased risk for overgrowth.[36]

Zebrowski et al. (1994) suggested that increased tissue levels of non-sulfated glycosaminoglycans can occur with cyclosporin exposure, possibly contributing to the occurrence of increased connective tissue matrix.[17] Keratinocyte growth factor plays a role in tissue repair and regeneration, proliferation and differentiation of epithelial cells. It inhibits the expression of epithelial cell specific collagenase-1 thereby causing excessive accumulation of extracellular matrix, as seen in gingival overgrowth. Levels of keratinocyte growth factor are increased in cyclosporin-induced gingival overgrowth, thereby suggesting a role in its pathogenesis.[37] A higher perlecan, a basement membrane proteoglycan, expression might be related to the increase in subepithelial and vascular basement membranes seen in cyclosporin-induced gingival overgrowth.[38]

Cyclosporin regulates the cytokine expression in the gingival tissues. It upregulates IL-6, which may play an important role in the pathogenesis of gingival overgrowth. Cyclosporin-induced gingival overgrowth tissue contains higher levels of IL-6 as compared to the normal or inflamed tissue. In a study, it was observed that levels of IL-1β increased in the overgrown tissue as compared to the normal or inflamed tissue, however this increase was not statistically significant.[39]

Growth factors have been studied as one obvious target for cyclosporin-induced gingival overgrowth, and their activation may play an important role in pathogenesis. Platelet derived growth factor acts as a major mitogen and chemoattractant for fibroblast proliferation and synthesis of glycosaminoglycans, fibronectin and collagen. Increased gingival levels of platelet-derived growth factor-B may be responsible for promoting fibroblast proliferation and production of extracellular matrix constituents in gingival overgrowth. The macrophage is now recognized as the major mediator of connective tissue turnover, maintenance and repair through release of specialized cytokines (platelet-derived growth factor-β).[17] Epidermal growth factor stimulates migration of cells, production of proteinase, proliferation of fibroblasts, synthesis of fibroblast collagen and hyaluronan and expression of certain proteolytic enzymes in the fibroblasts including MMP-1 and MMP-3. Cyclosporin therapy leads to higher mRNA and protein expression of epidermal growth factor and its receptor.[40]

Plaque-induced gingival inflammation augments the severity of cyclosporin-induced gingival overgrowth. Hence, proper oral hygiene can be expected to minimize the severity by eliminating the inflammatory component of the lesion.[41]

The relationship between the incidence and severity of cyclosporin-induced gingival overgrowth and various drug pharmacokinetic variables is controversial. It has been postulated that a certain threshold concentration of the drug is required to induce the gingival reaction and that increased levels of the drug above this threshold do not increase the severity of the lesion. Local concentrations of the drug in saliva, gingival crevicular fluid or plaque could also influence the expression and pathogenesis of the drug. Because of its lipophilic nature, the free fraction of plasma cyclosporin may enter saliva by passive diffusion. There is a positive correlation between cyclosporin concentration in stimulated saliva and the extent of gingival overgrowth.[42]

The age and sex may be additional factors that may influence the incidence and severity of cyclosporin-induced gingival overgrowth. An increase in the biologically active form of testosterone has been found in the overgrown tissues of patients suffering from drug-induced gingival overgrowth. Such alterations of androgen metabolism may account for the increased propensity for cyclosporin-induced gingival overgrowth in children and adolescents.[42]

Another mechanism that may be involved in the pathogenesis of cyclosporin-induced gingival overgrowth is the influence of the drug on sodium and calcium flux of the gingival fibroblasts. The production of collagenase is modulated by calcium influx and that once collagenase production is altered, fibroblasts of affected patients produce an inactive form of collagenase or a smaller amount of collagenase.[43] In either case, there would be an unregulated increase in gingival connective tissue volume. Therefore, the action of these various drugs on the sodium and calcium ion influx may prove to be the key to understanding why three dissimilar drugs have a common side effect on a secondary target tissue such as gingival connective tissue.[41]

Calcium Channel Blockers

Calcium channel blockers or calcium antagonists are a group of drugs specifically developed to assist in the management of cardiovascular conditions including hypertension, angina pectoris, coronary artery disease and cardiac arrhythmias.

Classification[20]

Calcium channel blockers can be classified as:

- Dihydropyridines: Nifedipine, Nicardipine, Isradipine, Amlodipine, Nitrendipine, Felodipine.

- Phenylakylamine derivatives: Verapamil

- Benzothiazine derivatives: Diltiazem

Mechanism of Action

Calcium channel blockers act by inhibiting calcium ion influx across the cell membrane of cardiac and smooth muscle cells, thereby interfering or blocking mobilization of calcium intracellularly. Depending on the specific agent, this results in dilatation of coronary arteries and arterioles, as well as decreased myocardial contractility and oxygen demand. Since 1978, dihydropyridines have been used to treat angina pectoris, postmyocardial syndrome and hypertension.

Pharmacokinetics

All calcium channel blockers are absorbed 90-100% orally, peak occurring at 1-3 hours (except amlodidpine: 6-9 hours). The oral bioavailability of calcium channel blockers is incomplete with marked inter and intraindividual variations because of the first pass metabolism. They are highly plasma protein bound (maximum: felodipine-99%, minimum: dilitiazem-80%) and have extensive tissue distribution. The half-life ranges from 2-6 hours except for amlodipine which has an exceptionally long half-life. They are 90% metabolized in the liver and excreted in the urine.[20]

The primary undesirable side effect of the calcium channel blockers results from excessive vasodilation, which manifests as facial flushing, dizziness, headache and edema. Other side effects like constipation, nausea, bradycardia are also seen.[20] Ramon et al. was the first to report a calcium channel blocker (nifedipinc)-induced gingival overgrowth in 1984. Gingival overgrowth is associated with five other agents in this class including amlodipine, felodipine, diltiazem, nitrendipine and verapamil. Another agent in this group, oxodipine, has been associated with gingival overgrowth in dogs and rats. A wider prevalence rate was observed from nifedipine as compared the other drugs.[17]

Nifedipine

Nifedipine is a dihyropyridine calcium channel blocker. It is used in the management of angina pectoris and hypertension. It is also used as an alternate drug for premature labor. It has a bioavailability of 30-60% and a half-life of 2-5 hours.

Gingival overgrowth associated with nifedipine therapy was first reported by Lederman et al in 1984.[19] The hyperplasia appears shortly after the start of the therapy and decreases on withdrawal of the drug. The prevalence rate of gingival overgrowth in patients on nifedipine therapy is 15-85%[43] Differing indices of overgrowth, differing populations, dosage and duration of medication are possible explanations for the differences between studies. It seems probable that the actual prevalence is toward the lower end of the range as the drug is widely prescribed around the world.[30]

Ishida et al. (1995) and Nishikawa et al. (1991) reported that a minimum blood level of 800 ng/ml of nifedipine resulted in gingival overgrowth in a rat model and that the degree of overgrowth depended on increased concentrations above this threshold value. Despite the absence of any evidence corroborating a relationship between nifedipine dose and overgrowth in humans, it is reasonable to suggest that a trough or threshold level must precede the onset of gingival enlargement. This value may differ depending on host (responder) susceptibility and sensitivity.[17]

Ellis et al (1993) showed nifedipine concentrates in the gingival crevicular fluid up to 90 times the serum concentration and, of the 9 patients examined, nifedipine could be found in the crevicular fluid of 5 patients with gingival overgrowth and two of the 'non-responders'.[17]

Clinical Features

1. The interdental papillae are initially affected, becoming enlarged and resulting in a lobulated or nodular morphology (Fig 6).[44]

2. These effects are limited to the attached and marginal gingiva, and are more frequently observed anteriorly, especially on the facial surfaces.[44]

3.   The enlarged gingiva may extend coronally and partially or completely obscure the teeth, presenting esthetic and functional difficulties for affected patients.

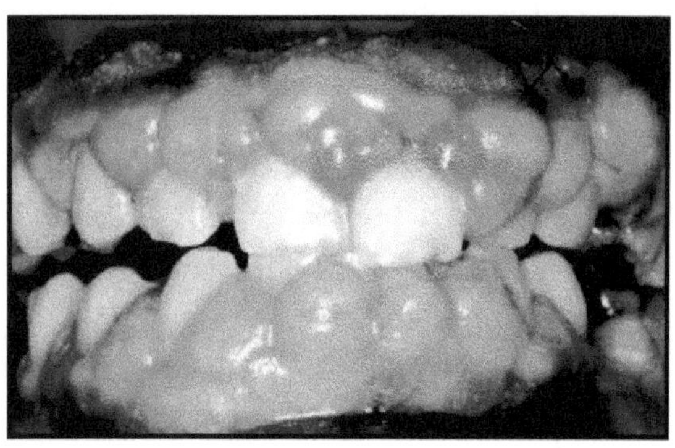

Fig 6. Calcium channel blocker-induced gingival enlargement.

4.   It does not appear to affect edentulous areas.

5.   Nifedipine-induced gingival enlargement has been reported around dental implants.[17]

6.   The enlarged gingival tissues are often accompanied by inflammatory changes associated with poor plaque control. As the tissues become progressively larger, plaque control becomes more difficult.

7.   Gingival enlargement is greater in patients who are medicated with both cyclosporin and calcium channel-blocking drugs.[32,33,34,35] It has been suggested

that combined therapy may increase the prevalence of the condition but not the severity and that it is a significant risk factor for progression and recurrence of the lesion after treatment.

Histologic Features [17, 19]

1. The epithelium exhibits parakeratosis, proliferation and elongation of the rete ridges, which extend some distance into the lamina propria.

2. There may be a ten-fold increase in epithelial width (normally 0.3 to 0.5 mm).

3. Thickening of the spinous cell layer, slight to moderate hyperkeratosis, fibroblastic proliferation and fibrosis of the lamina propria is also seen (Fig 7).

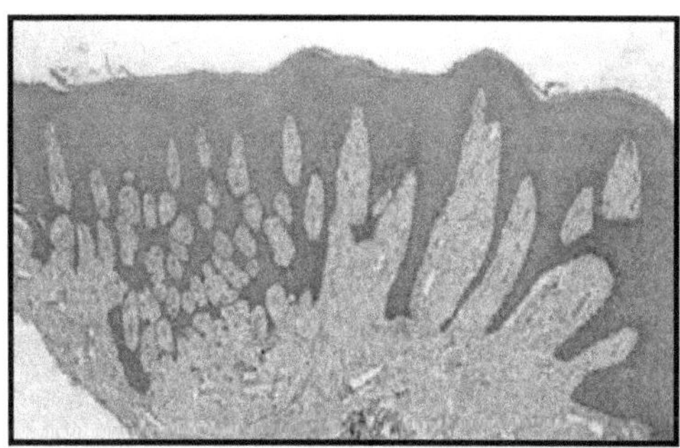

Fig 7. Histological section of calcium channel blocker-induced gingival enlargement

4.   The underlying connective tissue comprises of a diffuse mixture of dense collagen with varying amounts of ground substance.

5.   Inflammatory cells are present in the connective tissue, mainly plasma cells and lymphocytes.

6.   These changes could be accompanied by increased capillary vascularity and slight perivascular inflammation.

Other Calcium Channel Blockers

Amlodipine

Amlodipine is a dihydropyridine calcium channel blocker that acts by decreasing myocardial contractility and oxygen demand and that dilates coronary arteries and arterioles. It is used to treat angina and hypertension. Pharmacokinetically, it is the most distinct dihydropyridine. It has complete but slow absorption, peak is achieved after 6-9 hours. Because of less extensive and less variable first pass metabolism, its oral bioavailability is higher and more consistent.[20] It has a long half-life (35-50 hours). Although it is administered in the dosage of 5-10 mg/day, gingival enlargement could be a side effect.[30] Compared to phenytoin, cyclosporin or nifedipine, amlodipine has a higher volume of distribution and a longer half-life, which may account for the 200-fold increase in the gingival crevicular concentration compared to the plasma concentrations. This increased concentration could account for the gingival enlargement.

In a report of three cases of associated gingival overgrowth, amlodipine was detected in the gingival crevicular fluid of each individual, all of whom were long-term recipients of the medication. Gingival overgrowth began two to three months after starting the medication at 5-10 mg/day and the authors felt these changes were compounded by the patient's existing periodontal condition.[45]

Histologically, the collagenous stroma appears loose and filled with plump active fibroblasts with lots of ground substances. The overlying epithelium shows acantholytic changes.[46]

Nitrendipine

It is a long acting dihydropyridine used for angina pectoris and hypertension. Brown et al. (1990) reported the first case of gingival overgrowth induced by nitrendipine. Gingival enlargement was noticed within two months of the usage of the drug. They stated that nitrendipine-induced gingival overgrowth is like phenytoin-induced gingival overgrowth.

Histologically, the connective tissue shows an increase in vascularity and a loose matrix. [46]

Felodipine

It is a dihydropyridine used for arterial hypertension. It differs from nifedipine in having greater vascular selectivity, larger tissue distribution and a half-life of 12-18 hours. The extended-release preparation is suitable for once daily preparation.[20]

Only a few cases of gingival overgrowth ascribed to felodipine are reported in detail in the literature. Gingival overgrowth began soon after the commencement of felodipine therapy. Given the wide prescription of this drug it is assumed that the prevalence of gingival overgrowth associated with this drug is low.[30]

Histologically, a conspicuous increase of fibrous connective tissue, as well as an inflammatory infiltrate and hyperplasia of the overlying epithelium are seen. More glycosaminoglycans are noted in the extracellular substance than with nifedipine. Water-binding to these molecules is thought to be a factor in gingival enlargement.[46]

Oxodipine

It causes a dose dependent, purely fibroblastic proliferation without any inflammatory cell infiltrate.[46]

Manidipine

Manidipine hydrochloride (manidipine), a second-generation calcium channel blocker was launched in 1990. It has advantages of milder and longer action, weaker side effects as compared to the first-generation calcium channel blockers. Ikawa et al (2002) reported on a patient with severe gingival overgrowth who was on manidipine and carteolol for treatment of hypertension. Without the change or cessation of drug, standard periodontal therapy resulted in disappearance of gingival overgrowth.

Verapamil

Verapamil is a phenylalkylamine derivative calcium channel blocker. Verapamil is used to treat angina pectoris, essential hypertension and supra-ventricular arrhythmias. It has a half-life of 4-6 hours and a bioavailability of 15-30%.[20]

Its action is slower than that of nifedipine and this is thought to explain the lower prevalence rate of 4% of gingival overgrowth.47 Low therapeutic doses (<100 g/l) do not result in gingival enlargement. However higher doses (100-600 g/l) do cause gingival enlargement, which often begins in the maxillary and mandibular anterior interdental regions.[46] The early reports of gingival overgrowth associated with this drug began in the mid-1980s. The prevalence of verapamil-induced overgrowth appears to be very low. Although Steele et al. (1994) reported a 19% prevalence rate of gingival enlargement among verapamil patients, Miller and Damm (1992) found this side effect in only 4% of verapamil subjects examined. They could only find three cases in their review of 5000 dental patients seen over three years. They found only 24 patients taking verapamil for more than a year and only one of these patients showed gingival overgrowth.[47]

Histologically, increased extracellular ground substance and more fibroblasts containing sulphated mucopolysaccharides as secretory granules are seen.[46] Incubation of fibroblasts in the presence of verapamil showed reduced protein and collagen synthesis.[19] These findings would suggest that verapamil affects the proliferation of selected fibroblast subpopulations and alters the balance between regeneration and degradation.[44]

Prevention and treatment are directed at meticulous plaque control, scaling and root planing, antiseptic rinses and surgical excision if required.47 Discontinuance of the medication is the only absolute treatment for associated gingival symptoms, which may resolve within 15 days. Because of the relatively low apparent risk of gingival overgrowth with this agent, it has been used as a treatment alternative to other calcium channel blockers.[17]

Dilitiazem

Diltiazem is a benzothiazine derivative calcium channel blocker. It used in the management of angina pectoris and hypertension. It is a less potent vasodilator than nifedipine and verapamil and has a half-life of 5-6 hours and a bioavailability of 40-60%.[20]

Steele et al. (1994) reported a 21% prevalence rate of gingival enlargement among patients on dilitiazem. The medication may act directly or indirectly on calcium dependent mechanisms to alter collagen homeostasis and adversely affect the gingival tissues. The clinical and histological features of diltiazem-associated overgrowth are like those observed with phenytoin and other calcium channel blockers.[17] In a case report by Giustiani S et al (1987), a heart patient who developed gingival overgrowth because of verapamil therapy, discontinuance of the drug resulted in resolution. However, the overgrowth recurred in 24 days being more prominent around the labial surfaces of anterior teeth, when an alternate medication, diltiazem (240 mg/day), was administered, suggesting a similar mode of action at the gingival level.[17,30]

Pathogenesis

Despite unrelated pharmaceutical effects, the calcium channel blockers and phenytoin have a common mechanism of action related to the ability of each of these agents to affect calcium metabolism. As mentioned earlier, among the factors that may influence the pathogenesis of drug-associated gingival overgrowth are age, genetic predisposition, pharmacokinetic variables, alterations in gingival connective tissue homeostasis and drug effects on growth factors.

There does not appear to be a clear relationship between the dose of nifedipine and gingival enlargement.[17]

Fujii et al. (1994) tested the effect of calcium channel blockers on cell proliferation, DNA synthesis and collagen synthesis on gingival fibroblasts from human nifedipine responders and nonresponders. Cells were tested with nifedipine, diltiazem, verapamil and nicardipine in vitro. Responder fibroblasts tended toward greater cellular proliferation rates, DNA synthesis and collagen synthesis compared to the cells from nonresponders.

Nifedipine may interfere with calcium transport, intracellular calcium uptake and calcium-dependent processes. These agents may reduce cytosolic calcium levels in gingival fibroblasts and T cells, thus interfering with T cell proliferation or activation and collagen synthesis by gingival fibroblasts.43

Lucas et al. and Jones et al. (1985) suggested that gingival overgrowth results from overproduction of extracellular ground substance characterized by increased presence of sulphated-mucopolysaccharides (glycosaminoglycan) and collagen and abundant active fibroblasts.

McKevitt et al. (1995) used fibroblasts from responders and nonresponders to study the effect of phenotypic differences in growth, matrix synthesis and response to nifedipine. The responder cells presented increased growth potential and produced greater levels of protein and collagen than did nonresponder cells.[17]

Combination Therapy

The most common combination of drugs that cause gingival overgrowth is cyclosporin and nifedipine. Nifedipine is used frequently to treat hypertension which may be primary or secondary to cyclosporin nephrotoxicity. A significant increase in the incidence of gingival overgrowth has been described in renal transplant patients taking nifedipine as well as cyclosporin compared with those taking cyclosporin alone (51 per cent compared with 8 per cent).[30] Some investigators believed that increased prevalence and severity of gingival overgrowth in renal patients taking both drugs was unrelated to local factors and pharmacological parameters. They indicated a trend for HLA-A19 positive patients to show signs of gingival overgrowth, suggesting an underlying genetic susceptibility.[34]

Further studies of renal and cardiac transplant patients have suggested that while the incidence of clinically significant gingival overgrowth may be similar, the severity of overgrowth appears to be significantly greater in those receiving both cyclosporin and nifedipine.[32] These patients had significantly higher gingival overgrowth scores, probing depths and a greater need for surgery.

Verapamil and cyclosporin interactions have also been investigated in renal transplant patients. While there was an increased prevalence and severity of gingival overgrowth in patients taking both drugs, it was not significant. The dosage of either drug was unrelated to overgrowth. The authors concluded that verapamil was having no augmenting effect on either the severity or the prevalence of the gingival overgrowth.[17]

Other Drugs

Erythromycin

A single case of gingival overgrowth has been associated with the use of erythromycin in a young boy. The condition resolved on withdrawal of the drug and returned upon repeat challenge.[48]

Risk Factors

There is a variable gingival response in patients taking drugs like immunosuppressants, calcium channel blockers and anti-epileptics. Different patients show variability in the extent and severity of the gingival changes. The term ''clinically significant overgrowth'' has been applied to those patients whose gingival changes require surgical intervention to restore gingival contour.[32] The various risk factors that have been elucidated for drug-induced gingival overgrowth are age and other demographic factors, drug variables, concomitant medication, periodontal variables and genetic factors (Fig 8).[49]

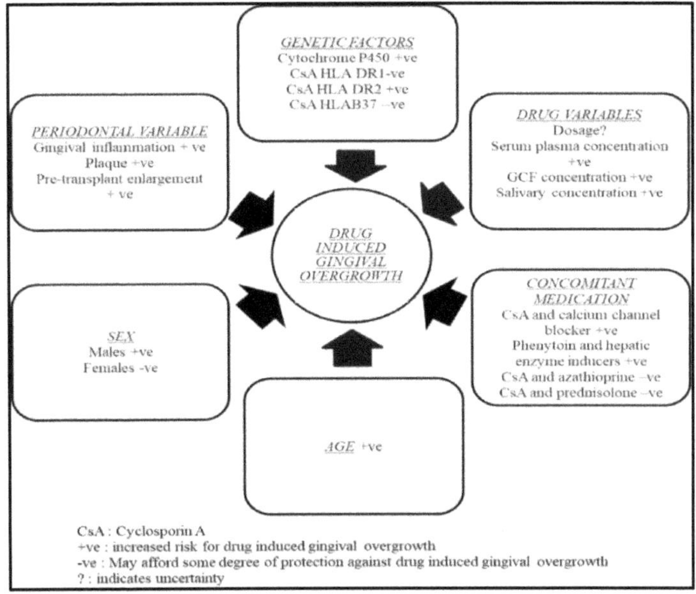

Fig 8. Overview of identified factors contributing to drug induced gingival overgrowth

Age and Demographic Factors

Age has been considered an important risk factor for drug-induced gingival overgrowth with reference to phenytoin and cyclosporin.[42] A community-based study reported that the combination of younger age and poor oral hygiene seemed to predispose to the severest level of gingival involvement.[49]

Age is not an applicable risk factor for the calcium channel blockers since the use of these drugs is usually confined to the middle aged and older adults. However, in patients medicated with both cyclosporin and calcium channel blockers, age has been identified as a risk factor.[50]

The differences in the prevalence of the overgrowth induced by these different drugs reflects the different age groups at which they are targeted, [53] phenytoin being targeted mainly at the young, calcium channel blockers at the post middle aged and cyclosporin across a broad range of ages. One possible explanation for this association may reside with an interaction between circulating androgens and gingival fibroblasts. Such cells can readily metabolize testosterone to the active metabolite 5 α-dihydrotestosterone. Phenytoin enhances this metabolism and excised tissue from both cyclosporin and nifedipine-induced gingival overgrowth exhibits a similar increase in androgen metabolism.[51] Circulating androgen levels will be higher in adolescents and teenagers, and the active metabolite could act on sub-populations of gingival fibroblasts and cause either an increase in collagen synthesis and/or a decrease in collagenase activity.

Other Demographic Variables

Gender and race are not important risk factors for the expression of drug-induced gingival overgrowth.[23]

Some cyclosporin studies report higher gingival overgrowth scores in males[49] but differences were not statistically significant. Males were also shown to be 3 times more likely than females to develop clinically significant gingival changes when medicated with calcium channel blockers.[52] Males have a lower serum threshold above which overgrowth occurs and the gingival changes are more severe as compared to females. This could be attributed to existing periodontal factors, pharmacological variables or a hormonal co-factor.[49]

Drug Variables

The relationship between the extent and severity of gingival overgrowth and a variety of drug variables (i.e., dose, duration, serum and salivary concentrations) remains an area of controversy.

Drug dosage tends to be a poor predictor of the gingival changes.[29] It would be appropriate to relate dose to the patient's body weight to obtain a more meaningful interpretation of dosage and its relationship to gingival overgrowth.

Studies investigating the relationship between serum concentrations of the implicated drug and the expression of gingival overgrowth have shown that both phenytoin and calcium channel blockers obtain steady state therapeutic drug levels at 7–10 days after the initiation of therapy. Thus, for these two drugs a serum sample at any time point is likely to be a true reflection of the drug's concentration.

The type of cyclosporin preparation may have some impact on the development of gingival overgrowth in organ transplant patients. Gingival overgrowth was observed in 37% of the patients taking the cyclosporin solution, compared to 43% dosed with capsules. However, the solution patients showed an earlier onset of gingival changes and more extensive overgrowth than those medicated with capsules. In this study the different effects of the two cyclosporin preparations on the gingival tissues may be related to subsequent changes in the drug's pharmacokinetics, in particular bioavailability and time to maximum blood concentrations.[35]

Pallavi Sharma, Dwiti Thanawala,
Alankrita Chaudhary, Himani Sharma

Several studies have investigated whether salivary concentrations of these drugs are important determinants for gingival overgrowth. For phenytoin, some studies have reported that salivary concentrations are positively correlated with gingival overgrowth[23], whilst others have failed to confirm such a relationship.[54] It is possible that the concentration of phenytoin or its major metabolite (HPPH) present in saliva are not representative of those present at the site of action, that is, the gingival tissue itself. A positive correlation has been found between cyclosporin concentrations in stimulated saliva and the extent of gingival overgrowth.[42] Other studies, however, have reported a lack of correlation between unstimulated salivary cyclosporin levels and gingival overgrowth.[49] These conflicting findings may be explained by the fact that dental plaque may act as a reservoir for cyclosporin, which is then released by the actions of stimulated salivary flow.[55] Thus, whilst salivary samples are easy to collect, they may not be as useful an indicator for the development of gingival overgrowth.

Local concentrations of both phenytoin and the dihydropyridine class of calcium channel blockers in gingival crevicular fluid (GCF) have provided some useful insight into local tissue activity.[45,56] GCF concentrations of phenytoin do not appear to be related to the extent of gingival overgrowth.56 However, significant sequestration of both nifedipine and amlodipine has been observed in patients who exhibit significant gingival changes arising from these drugs.45 Despite the high levels of nifedipine sequestered in the GCF only the plasma concentration of nifedipine was identified as a risk factor for the severity of the gingival changes.

Other pharmacokinetic measures that may be more pertinent in relation to gingival overgrowth include bioavailability, degree of protein binding, volume of distribution, and an overall assessment of drug concentration in relation to time.

Concomitant Medication

Considerable body of evidence that the combination of nifedipine and cyclosporin in organ transplant patients produces more gingival overgrowth than if either drug was used singularly.[32,33,34,35] It has been suggested that combined therapy may increase the prevalence of the condition but not the severity and that it is a significant risk factor for progression and recurrence of the lesion after treatment.[57]

Pallavi Sharma, Dwiti Thanawala,
Alankrita Chaudhary, Himani Sharma

In adult organ transplant patients, dosages of both prednisolone and azathioprine appeared to afford the patients some degree of protection against the development of gingival overgrowth, whereas in children dosing with azathioprine did likewise. Other studies have shown that both azathioprine and prednisolone reduce the severity of drug-induced gingival overgrowth in organ transplant patients.[53] The so-called protective effect of these two drugs on gingival overgrowth may arise from their anti-inflammatory actions on plaque- gingival inflammation.

Phenytoin is metabolised (hydrolysed) in the liver by P450 enzymes to 5-(4-hydroxyphenyl)-5-phenylhydantoin (4-HPPH). This metabolite has been shown to induce gingival overgrowth in cats.[58] Anticonvulsants such as phenobarbitone, primidone and carbamazepine have been shown to induce hepatic P450 isoenzyme and if given in conjunction with phenytoin, it will increase serum concentrations of 4-HPPH. This may explain the increased prevalence of gingival overgrowth in patients receiving multiple anticonvulsant therapy.

Periodontal Variables

Plaque scores and gingival inflammation appear to exacerbate the expression of drug-induced gingival overgrowth, irrespective of the initiating drug.[29] Most of the evidence to support a relationship between bacterial plaque and gingival overgrowth has been derived from cross-sectional studies and it is not clear whether plaque is a contributory factor or a consequence of the gingival changes.[49]

The effect of an oral hygiene programme on cyclosporin-induced gingival overgrowth was examined in a longitudinal trial.49 Both the case and the control group developed significant gingival changes over the 6-month post-transplant investigation period, although the magnitude of the changes in the oral hygiene group was less marked. Oral hygiene therapy, whilst of some benefit to the patients, failed to prevent the development of gingival overgrowth. It would be reasonable to suggest that proper oral hygiene might minimize the severity of cyclosporin-induced gingival overgrowth, possibly by eliminating the inflammatory component of the lesion but improved oral hygiene would not prevent the overgrowth.

A study evaluating the impact of a patient's periodontal condition prior to organ transplantation on the development of gingival overgrowth post-transplant showed that patients who exhibited a hyperplastic gingivitis prior to transplant were highly likely to develop severe gingival changes post-transplant.[59] This would suggest a susceptibility of the gingival tissues (or fibroblasts) to both plaque-induced inflammatory changes and cyclosporin.

Periodontal variables in particular plaque and gingival inflammation are also important risk factors for the expression of gingival overgrowth attributable to the calcium channel blockers. It is noted that gingival changes are more pronounced in patients taking nifedipine for cardiovascular disorders compared to those taking these drugs whilst under haemodialysis.[49]

Genetic Factors

Fibroblast heterogeneity remains one of the key factors used to explain the variable response of the gingival tissues to the various drug-induced gingival overgrowth. However, it has limited clinical value in identifying patients at risk, as there is no clinical marker of gingival fibroblast phenotype. A genetic predisposition could influence the metabolism of phenytoin, cyclosporin and nifedipine, since all three drugs are metabolised by the hepatic cytochrome P450 enzymes. Cytochrome P450 genes exhibit considerable polymorphism which results in inter-individual variation in enzyme activity, which may influence the patient's serum and tissue concentrations and hence their gingival response.

The one genetic marker that has been investigated in relation to drug-induced gingival overgrowth is the human lymphocyte antigen expression. Investigation of this marker has been confined to the organ transplant patients since their HLA phenotype is determined prior to transplantation. Several studies have reported on the relationship between HLA expression and the incidence of drug-induced gingival overgrowth.[34,57]

A study reported that patients who expressed HLA-DR1 are afforded some degree of protection against gingival overgrowth whilst HLA-DR2 may increase the development of this unwanted effect.[36] A trend towards an increased presence of HLA-A19 antigen has also been reported although the relationship was not significant after correction for multiple significance testing.[34] To date only HLA-B37 has been identified as a significant risk factor after correction for the effect of multiple significance testing and these patients are protected in some way from the effects of gingival overgrowth.[50] The concept of molecular mimicry in the wider field of periodontal disease or an effect on lymphocyte function[36] have been postulated as the mechanisms that may tie HLA antigens to gingival overgrowth.

Indices

The gingival overgrowth indexes proposed in the literature are diversified from the simplest to the most elaborate ones. Some of the indices used for assessing gingival overgrowth are as follows:

<u>Degree of gingival enlargement can be scored according to Bokenkamp & Bohnhorst, 1994[33]</u>

- Grade 0 - No sign of gingival enlargement.

- Grade 1 - Enlargement confined to interdental papillae.

- Grade 2 - Enlargement involves interdental papillae and marginal gingiva.

- Grade 3 - Enlargement covers three quarters / more of crown.

<u>Degree of gingival hyperplasia according to modified index by Angelopoulos and Goaz, 1972[60]</u>

- Grade 0 - No hyperplasia normal gingiva.

- Grade 1 - Minimal hyperplasia: less than 2mm increase in size and the gingiva covers cervical third or less than the anatomic crown.

- Grade 2 - Moderate hyperplasia: 2 to 4 mm increase in size and/or gingiva extends into the middle third of the anatomic crown.

- Grade 3 - Severe hyperplasia: nodular growth, greater than 4mm increase in size and/or gingiva covers more than two thirds of the tooth crown.

<u>Gingival overgrowth index of McGaw et al, 1987[60]</u>

- Grade 0 - No overgrowth, feather edged gingival margin.

- Grade 1 - Blunting of gingival margin.

- Grade 2 - Moderate gingival overgrowth (one- third crown length).

- Grade 3 - Marked gingival overgrowth (more than one- third crown length).

<u>Clinical index for drug-induced gingival overgrowth by Ingles et al, 1999[60]</u>

- Grade 0

1: No overgrowth, firm adaptation of the attached gingiva to the underlying alveolar bone.

2: There is slight stippling, but no granular appearance or a slight granular appearance.

3: A knife edged papilla is present towards the occlusal surface.

4: There is no increase in density or size of the gingiva.

- Grade 1

1: Early overgrowth, as evidenced by an increased density of the gingiva, with marked stippling and granular appearance.

2: The tip of the papilla is rounded.

3: The probing depth is ≤ 3 mm.

- Grade 2

1: Moderate overgrowth, manifested by an increase in the size of the papilla and/or rolled gingival margins.

2: The contour of the gingiva is still concave or straight.

3: Gingival enlargement has a bucco-lingual dimension of upto 2 mm measured from the tip of the papilla outward.

4: The probing depth is ≤ 6 mm.

5: The papilla is somewhat retractable.

- Grade 3

1: Marked overgrowth represented by encroachment of the gingiva on the clinical crown.

2: The contour of the gingival margin is convex rather than concave.

3: Gingival enlargement has a buccolingual dimension $\geq$ 3 mm or more, measured from the tip of the papilla outward.

4: The probing depth is > 6 mm.

5: The papilla is clearly retractable.

- Grade 4

1: Severe overgrowth characterized by a profound thickening of the gingiva.

2: A large percentage of the clinical crown is covered.

3: Gingival enlargement has a buccolingual dimension $\leq$ 3 mm, measured from the tip of the papilla outward, the probing depth is > 6 mm and the papilla is clearly retractable.

This index describes gingival condition in buccolingual dimension and apico-coronal dimension or probing depth, texture and density of gingival tissues, shape, contour of the papilla (mesiodistally) and retractability.

Ellis et al, 2001[61] described a photographic scoring method for DIGO, which is suitable for use in large scale population.

Prevention and Treatment

Effective treatment of a condition such as this generally focuses on correction of the aesthetic and/or functional problems that result and can be divided into either nonsurgical or surgical alternatives (Fig. 9).

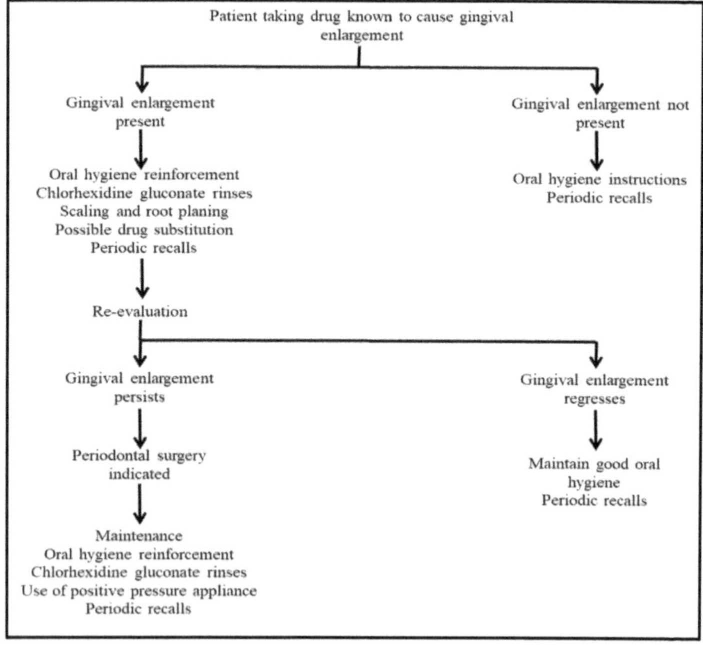

Fig 9. Decision tree in the treatment of DIGO

Non-Surgical Therapy

The primary aim of non-surgical therapy is to reduce the inflammatory component in the gingival tissues and thereby avoid the need for surgery. Ideally preventive programmes should be instituted before the initiation of the drug therapies implicated in drug-induced gingival overgrowth[25] However, for prospective transplant patients, this is often impractical as such patients are frequently too unwell for such measures to be instituted.

Given the significance of plaque and calculus as a risk factor for exacerbation of gingival overgrowth, initial periodontal therapy comprising comprehensive oral hygiene advice to ensure optimal home care along with regular professional debridement should be rendered. Although the exact role played by bacterial plaque in drug-induced gingival enlargement is unclear, there is evidence that good oral hygiene and frequent professional removal of plaque decreases the degree of the gingival enlargement present and improves overall gingival health.[29]

For some patients these measures alone could reduce the gingival overgrowth to acceptable levels, for others it could make surgical correction easier.[62] Local environmental factors that enhance plaque accumulation such as faulty restorations, broken teeth or carious lesions should be eliminated, and any fixed or removable prostheses should be designed to minimize plaque retention. Adequate plaque control may aid in preventing or retarding the recurrence of gingival enlargement in surgically treated cases.[63]

Antiseptic Mouthwashes

Adjunctive chemical plaque removal has also been used in the management of drug-induced gingival overgrowth. Animal studies have shown that regular application of a chlorhexidine solution to rats medicated with cyclosporin resulted in significantly less overgrowth than in control animals. In humans to date, chlorhexidine has only been evaluated in the management of phenytoin-induced gingival overgrowth, when regular use of this mouthwash helps to reduce the recurrence rate after surgery.[62]

Systemic Antibiotics

Short courses of azithromycin and metronidazole have been evaluated in the management of drug-induced gingival overgrowth. According to Glaude and Synder (1990), evidence suggests that a combination of oral hygiene reinforcement and systemic antibiotics may be beneficial.

Benefits of metronidazole on the gingival tissues result from a change in the subgingival biofilm and an associated reduction in tissue inflammation. There are two suggested mechanisms by which azithromycin may act: [62]

i.   By reducing concomitant bacterial infection and hence inflammation.

ii.   By increasing the phagocytic activity of gingival fibroblasts, thereby reversing the ability of cyclosporin to decrease collagen degradation.

Other Agents

Phenytoin may interfere with folic acid absorption and metabolism. There is some evidence that a folic acid mouthwash (1 mg/ml) may be efficacious in reducing the recurrence of phenytoin-induced gingival overgrowth and that a mouthwash is more effective than systemic administration. Patients with low baseline plasma and red blood cell folate levels show a greater gingival response to topical folic acid than patients with normal levels.[62]

Isotretinoin inhibits proliferation and collagen synthesis of fibroblasts.19 In a case report by Norris and Cunliffe (1987), it was observed that phenytoin-induced gingival overgrowth significantly reduced when the patient was treated with isotretinoin for her facial acne.

Positive pressure appliances have been recommended as a means of preventing or reducing the recurrence of gingival overgrowth. The appliance should be worn for 8 hours or more daily to prevent or reduce the tendency to recurrence.[17]

Changes in Medication

Ideally, the treatment of choice for drug-induced gingival overgrowth would be discontinuation of the associated medication after consulting the physician. Nevertheless, this approach is often not possible.25 Spontaneous remission of drug-induced gingival overgrowth has been shown to take place following a change in medication combined with presence of good oral hygiene.

Phenytoin

Other anticonvulsant agents have been associated with gingival overgrowth since occurrence of this side effect is considered infrequent compared with phenytoin and hence can substitute it.

Other agents include primadone, phenobarbital, mephentoin, ethytoin, ethosuximide, and valproic acid[19] and relatively newer drugs like vigabatrin, lomatrigine, gabapentin, sulthiame and topiramate.[30]

Cyclosporin

Discontinuation of cyclosporin has shown that the gingival overgrowth disappears completely 3-12 months after drug suspension. The conversion from cyclosporin to tacrolimus produces a resolution of the gingival overgrowth within the first month. Tacrolimus (also FK-506) is an immunosuppressive drug whose main use is after allogeneic organ transplant to reduce the activity of the patient's immune system and thus lower the risk of organ rejection. A study by Oliveira et al (2006) showed patients treated with tacrolimus a 17.9% prevalence of gingival overgrowth while in the group medicated with cyclosporin it was 38.1%.64 Also, cyclosporin but not tacrolimus, induces gingival overgrowth with an increase in the salivary levels of transforming growth factor – β1, epidermal growth factor and interleukin- 6.[65]

In adult organ transplant patients, dosages of both prednisolone and azathioprine appeared to afford the patients some degree of protection against the development of gingival overgrowth, whereas in children dosing with only azathioprine did likewise. This effect may arise from their anti-inflammatory actions on plaque-induced gingival inflammation.[53]

Calcium Channel Blockers

For patients on nifedipine, where the prevalence of gingival enlargement has been reported to be up to 44%, other calcium-channel blockers such as diltiazem and verapamil may be viable alternatives since the prevalence of gingival enlargement associated with those drugs is 20% and 4%, respectively. Regression of nifedipine-induced gingival overgrowth has been reported when the drug was substituted by isradipine, a dihydropyridine calcium channel blocker.[17] Also, consideration may be given to the use of another class of antihypertensive medications than calcium-channel blockers, none of which are known to induce gingival enlargement.[50]

Although discontinuing the use of nifedipine has resulted in gingival improvement within 1-week, appreciable response may require much longer. Reinstitution of nifedipine therapy following withdrawal has resulted in recurrence of the gingival overgrowth within 4 weeks.[17]

Surgical Therapy

If gingival enlargement persists, despite of maintenance of good oral hygiene as well as drug substitution, then definitive treatment involves surgical elimination of the excess gingival tissue through implementation of either the gingivectomy procedure or periodontal flap approach. The use of laser surgical therapy is also becoming more common in treatment of gingival overgrowth due to its advantages in postoperative haemostasis.4

Maintenance

Recurrence of drug-induced gingival enlargement is a reality in surgically treated cases. As stated previously, meticulous home care, chlorhexidine gluconate rinses and close 3-monthly maintenance and professional debridement following surgery will decrease the rate and the degree at which recurrence occurs. A hard, natural rubber fitted bite guard worn at night may also assist in the control of recurrence. Recurrence may occur as early as 3–6 months after the surgical treatment, but in general, surgical results are maintained for at least 12 months.[18]

5. Enlargements Associated with Systemic Diseases

Many systemic diseases lead to development of oral manifestations including gingival enlargement and these diseases and/or conditions can impact the periodontium by two different mechanisms: [2]

1. Magnification of an existing inflammation initiated by dental plaque. This group of diseases, conditioned enlargements include some hormonal conditions (e.g. pregnancy and puberty), nutritional diseases such as vitamin C deficiency, and some cases in which the systemic influence is not identified (nonspecific conditioned enlargement).

2. Manifestation of the systemic disease independently of the inflammatory status of the gingiva. This group will be described under systemic diseases causing gingival enlargement and neoplastic enlargement (gingival tumors).

Conditioned Enlargements

Conditioned enlargement occurs because of exaggeration or distortion of the gingival response to dental plaque by the systemic condition of the. Although bacterial plaque is essential for the initiation of this type of enlargement, the nature of clinical features is not entirely determined by dental plaque.[2]

The three types of conditioned gingival enlargement are

- Hormonal (pregnancy, puberty)

- Nutritional (associated with vitamin C deficiency)

- Allergic

Gingival Enlargement due to Hormonal Changes

Hormones are specific regulatory molecules that modulate reproduction, growth and development, maintenance of the internal environment, as well as energy production, utilization, and storage. Hormonal effects reflect physiological as well as pathological changes in almost all types of body tissues. Periodontal tissues have receptors for several hormones such as androgens, estrogen, and progesterone, thus systemic endocrine imbalances may influence the periodontal pathogenesis.[66]

Pallavi Sharma, Dwiti Thanawala,
Alankrita Chaudhary, Himani Sharma

During the reproductive years, there are continuing changes in the concentration of the gonadotrophins and ovarian hormones during the menstrual cycle (Fig 1). Estrogen and progesterone are steroid hormones produced by the ovaries during the menstrual cycle. The gonadotrophins follicle-stimulating hormone (FSH) and luteinizing hormone (LH) influence estrogen and progesterone to prepare the uterus for implantation of the egg.

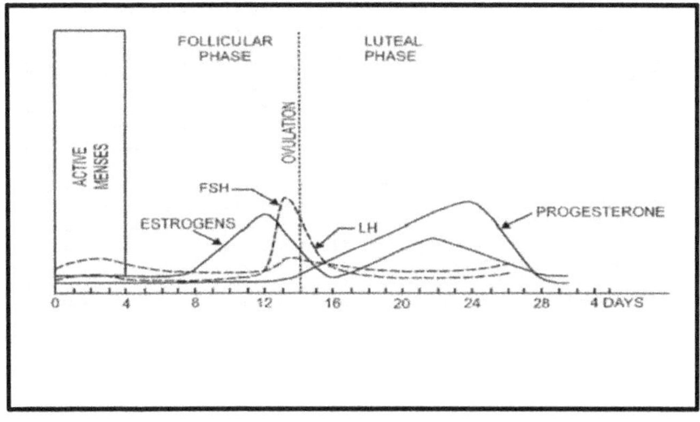

Fig 1. Female reproductive cycle

Estrogen and progesterone are responsible for physiological changes in women at specific stages of their life, starting in puberty. The influences of sex steroid hormones in the periodontium are multifarious.

Along with the microbial populations in the gingival sulcus, they affect the host by affecting the cellular (i.e., in the blood vessels, epithelium, and connective tissue) as well as the immune functions of the host.[67]

Puberty-Associated Gingival Enlargement

Gingival enlargement may occasionally be found during puberty in both male and female adolescents and in regions of plaque accumulation.

During puberty the production of sex hormones (estrogen and progesterone) increases and thereafter remains relatively constant post-puberty in a normal female reproductive phase. An increased prevalence of gingivitis without concurrent increase in the quantity of plaque has been noted.[68] There is alteration in the subgingival microflora with elevated bacterial counts and increased prevalence of certain microbial species such as Prevotella intermedia and Capnocytophaga species.[69] Prevotella intermedia possess the capability to substitute estrogen and progesterone for menadione (vitamin K) as an essential growth factor.[70] This may elucidate the association between augmented estrogen concentrations and the increased counts of Prevotella intermedia. Increase in Capnocytophaga species have been linked with an increase in the propensity to bleed.[69] Studies have shown proportionately elevated motile rods, spirochetes, Prevotella nigrescens and Prevotella intermedia in cases of puberty gingivitis.[68]

Clinical Features

Gingival enlargement during puberty has all the clinical features generally associated with chronic inflammatory gingival disease (Fig 2). It is the extent of enlargement and the tendency of recurrence in the presence of relatively little plaque deposits that distinguish puberty-associated gingival enlargement from uncomplicated chronic inflammatory gingival enlargement. It presents the following clinical features:

1. An increase in gingival inflammation in circumpubertal males and females without a concomitant increase in plaque levels.

2. It is seen in marginal gingivae and interdental papillae characterized by prominent bulbous interdental papillae

3. Nodular hyperplastic reaction of the gingiva may occur in regions where food debris, calculus, materia-alba, plaque are deposited.

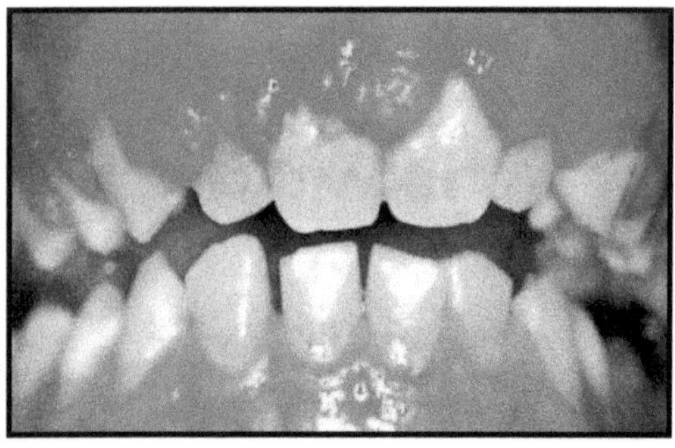

Fig 2. Puberty associated gingival enlargement

4.   The enlargement usually occurs on the facial gingivae with relatively unaltered lingual surfaces since the mechanical action of the tongue and the excursion of food avoids heavy accumulation of local irritants on the lingual surface.

5.   The inflamed tissues are erythematous and may be lobulated and retractable.

6.   Bleeding may occur with mastication or brushing.

Histologic Features

Histologically, the appearance is consistent with inflammatory hyperplasia with prominent edema and associated degenerative changes.[2,68]

Treatment

The enlargement may undergo spontaneous reduction post-puberty; however, it doesn't disappear until plaque and calculus are removed.2 Preventive rigorous oral hygiene is essential. Milder gingivitis cases respond well to scaling and root planing with regular reinforcements of oral hygiene instructions. Severe cases of gingivitis may require microbial culturing, antimicrobial mouthwashes, and antibiotic therapy. Frequent recall visits should be made. Involvement of a parent or caregiver with home-care procedures is suggested whenever possible.[68]

Pregnancy Associated Gingival Enlargement

During pregnancy there is an increase in levels of both progesterone and estrogen. Estrogen may regulate cellular proliferation, differentiation, and keratinization, while progesterone influences the permeability of the microvasculature, alters the rate and pattern of collagen production, and increases the metabolic breakdown of folate (necessary for tissue maintenance). These hormonal changes induce changes in vascular permeability leading to gingival edema and an increased inflammatory response to dental plaque.

The subgingival microbiota may also undergo changes, including an increase in Prevotella intermedia[2]

Etiologic Factors [68]

Alterations in the composition of subgingival plaque, maternal immunoresponsiveness and sex hormone concentrations create a myriad of responses in the periodontium.

Subgingival Plaque Composition

There is an alteration in the composition of subgingival plaque during pregnancy. During the second trimester there is an increase in gingivitis and gingival bleeding without an increase in plaque levels.70 Bacterial anaerobic-to-aerobic ratios also increase, including Bacteroides melaninogenicus, and Prevotella intermedia proportions (2.2 to 10.1%). There is also an increase in Porphyromonas gingivalis. Estradiol or progesterone substitute for menadione (vitamin K) as an essential growth factor for Prevotella intermedia. The percentage of Prevotella intermedia increase in the fourth month of pregnancy with an increase of hormones in saliva. Gingival inflammation is also more extensive in subjects who show more than 15% Prevotella intermedia in total colony forming units.

Pallavi Sharma, Dwiti Thanawala,
Alankrita Chaudhary, Himani Sharma

Maternal immunoresponsiveness

Alteration of immunocomponents during pregnancy results in changes in maternal immunoresponsiveness thereby showing increased susceptibility to gingival inflammation. During pregnancy, the gingival index is higher, but percentages of T3, T4 and B cells appear to decrease in peripheral blood and gingival tissues as compared to a control group. Other studies report decreased neutrophil chemotaxis, depression of cell-mediated immunity and phagocytosis, as well as a decreased T-cell response with elevated levels of progesterone.[71] High levels of progesterone during pregnancy affect the development of localized inflammation by down-regulation of IL-6 production, rendering the gingiva less efficient at resisting the inflammatory challenges produced by the bacteria.[68]

Ovarian hormones stimulate the production of prostaglandins, which act as immunosuppressants, thereby increasing gingival inflammation. Kinnby and colleagues found that high progesterone during pregnancy influenced plasminogen activator inhibitor type 2 (PAI-2) and disturbed the balance of the fibrinolytic system. Because PAI-2 serves as an important inhibitor of tissue proteolysis, the components of the fibrinolytic system may be involved in the development of pregnancy gingivitis.[72]

Sex hormone concentration

During pregnancy, plasma progesterone reaches levels of 100 ng/mL, 10 times the peak in the luteal phase of menses. Plasma estradiol levels may be 30 times higher than that during the reproductive cycle.

Specific estrogen and progesterone receptors are also present in the gingival tissues. A high concentration of sex hormones is observed in the gingival tissues, saliva, serum and crevicular fluid. The concentration of sex hormones increases in saliva from the first month of gestation, peaking in the ninth month along with increasing percentages of Prevotella intermedia. The number of gingival sites with bleeding and redness increases until one month postpartum. There is also evidence of sex hormone concentration in crevicular fluid, providing a growth media for periodontal pathogens.[68]

Types of Pregnancy-Associated Gingival Enlargement

Pregnancy-associated gingival enlargement may be marginal and generalized or may occur as single or multiple tumor-like masses.[2]

Marginal/ generalized enlargement

In 1877, Pinard recorded the first case of "pregnancy gingivitis." Pregnancy gingivitis is extremely common, occurring in approximately 30 to 75% of all pregnant women. It is characterized by erythema, edema, hyperplasia and increased bleeding. Histologically, the appearance is the same as gingivitis. Periodontal status prior to pregnancy also influences the progression or severity of the disease due to the fluctuation of the circulating hormones.[68]

Clinical Features

1. The enlargement is usually generalized and tends to be more prominent interproximally than on the facial and lingual surfaces.[2]

2. The anterior region of the mouth is more commonly affected.

3.   Anterior site inflammation may be exacerbated by increased mouth breathing, primarily in the third trimester from "pregnancy rhinitis". [68]

4.   The enlarged gingiva is bright red or magenta, soft and friable and has a smooth, shiny surface.[2]

5.   Bleeding occurs spontaneously or on slight provocation.

6.   Increased tissue edema may lead to increased pocket depths and relate to a transient tooth mobility.[68]

Tumour like enlargements

Pyogenic granulomas occur during pregnancy at a prevalence rate of 0.2 to 9.6%. The "pregnancy tumor" or "pregnancy epulis" are clinically and histologically indistinguishable from pyogenic granulomas occurring in women who are not pregnant or in men.68 The so-called pregnancy tumor is not a neoplasm, it is an inflammatory response to bacterial plaque and is modified by the patient's condition. They appear most commonly during the second or third month of pregnancy[2]

Clinical Features [2,68]

1.   The gingiva is the most common site involved (approximately 70% of all cases), followed by tongue and lips, buccal mucosa and palate.[73]

2.   It is a superficial lesion associated with poor oral hygiene and ordinarily does not invade the underlying bone.

3.   The lesion appears as a discrete, mushroom like, flattened spherical mass that protrudes from the gingival margin or more commonly from the interdental papillae of maxillary anterior teeth.

4.   It tends to expand laterally and pressure from the tongue and the cheek perpetuates its flattened appearance (Fig 3).

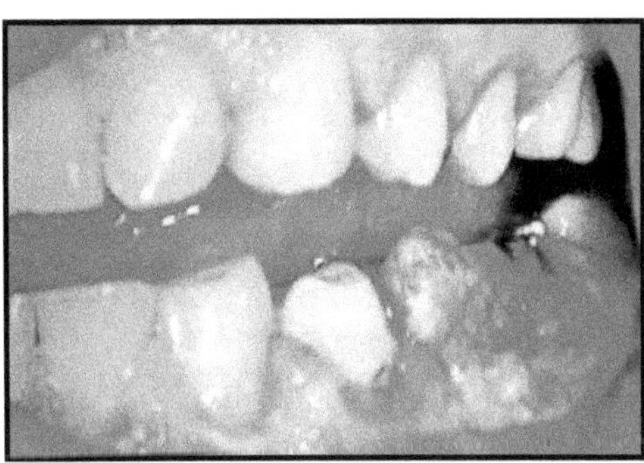

Fig 3. Pregnancy-associated gingival enlargement.

5. The color ranges from purplish red to deep blue, depending on the vascularity of the lesion and the degree of venous stasis.

6. It has a smooth, glistening surface that often exhibits numerous deep red, pinpoint markings.

7. The consistency is usually semi firm, but it may have various degrees of softness and friability.

8. It may be sessile or pedunculated base.

9. It usually grows rapidly, bleeds easily, and become hyperplastic and nodular.

10. It is usually painless unless its size and shape foster accumulation of debris under its margin or interfere with occlusion, in which case, painful ulceration may occur.

Histologic Features[2] (Fig 4)

Gingival enlargement in pregnancy is called an angiogranuloma. Both marginal and tumor like enlargements consist of a central mass of connective tissue, with numerous diffusely arranged, newly formed and engorged capillaries lined by cuboid endothelial cells, as well as a moderately fibrous stroma with varying degrees of edema and chronic inflammatory infiltrate. The stratified squamous epithelium is thickened, with prominent rete pegs and some degree of intracellular and extracellular edema, prominent intercellular bridges and leukocytic infiltration.

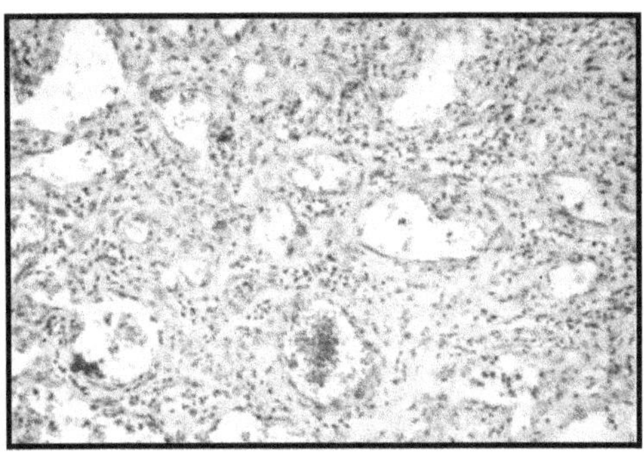

Fig 4. Histological section of pregnancy-associated gingival enlargement

Treatment [2]

Although spontaneous reduction in the size of gingival enlargement commonly follows the termination of pregnancy, complete elimination of the residual inflammatory lesion requires the removal of all plaque deposits and factors that favor its accumulation. Elimination of local irritants early in pregnancy is a preventive measure against gingival disease. In pregnancy, excision of the gingiva enlargement without complete elimination of local irritants is followed by recurrence of gingival enlargement.

Gingival lesions in pregnancy should be treated as soon as they are detected, although not necessarily by surgical means. Scaling and root planing procedures and adequate oral hygiene measures may reduce the size of the enlargement. Gingival enlargements do shrink after pregnancy, but they usually do not disappear. After pregnancy, the entire mouth should be reevaluated, a full set of radiographs taken, and the necessary treatment undertaken. Lesions should be removed surgically during pregnancy only if they interfere with mastication or produce an esthetic disFig.ment that the patient wishes to be removed.

In pregnancy, the emphasis should be on

1) Preventing gingival disease before it occurs.

2) Treating existing gingival disease before it worsens.

Every pregnant woman should be scheduled for periodic dental visits, the importance of which, in the prevention of serious periodontal disturbances, should be stressed.

Pallavi Sharma, Dwiti Thanawala,
Alankrita Chaudhary, Himani Sharma

Vitamin C Deficiency-Associated Gingival Enlargement

Although some nutritional deficiencies can significantly exacerbate the response of the gingiva to plaque bacteria, the precise role of nutrition in the initiation or progression of periodontal diseases remains to be elucidated. While there is paucity of information available regarding the effects of a specific, single nutritional deficiency on human periodontal tissues, severe vitamin C deficiency or scurvy has been one of the earliest nutritional deficiencies to be examined in the oral cavity[9]

In 1749, the Scottish surgeon James Lind discovered that citrus foods helped prevent scurvy. Since then studies have shown that low levels of plasma vitamin C are associated with some degree of gingivitis and periodontitis.19 Even though scurvy is unusual in areas with an adequate food supply, certain populations on restricted diets (e.g. infants from low socio-economic families) are at a risk of developing this condition.74 There are suggestions that lack of vitamins A, B2 and vitamin B12 complex may also be associated with changes in the gingiva.[1]

Clinical Features [2,19]

Enlargement of the gingiva is generally included in classic descriptions of scurvy. It is important to recognize that such enlargement is essentially a conditioned response to bacterial plaque. Acute vitamin C deficiency does not of itself cause gingival inflammation, but it does cause hemorrhage, collagen degeneration and edema of the gingival connective tissue. These changes modify the response of the gingiva to plaque to the extent that the normal defensive reaction is inhibited, and the extent of the inflammation is exaggerated. The combined effect of acute vitamin C deficiency and inflammation produces the massive gingival enlargement observed in scurvy.

1. Gingival enlargement in vitamin C deficiency is marginal and exaggerated by poor oral hygiene (Fig 5).

2. The gingiva becomes soft and friable, spongy, tender, boggy, bluish red in color (particularly the interdental papilla) and has a smooth, shiny surface.

Pallavi Sharma, Dwiti Thanawala,
Alankrita Chaudhary, Himani Sharma

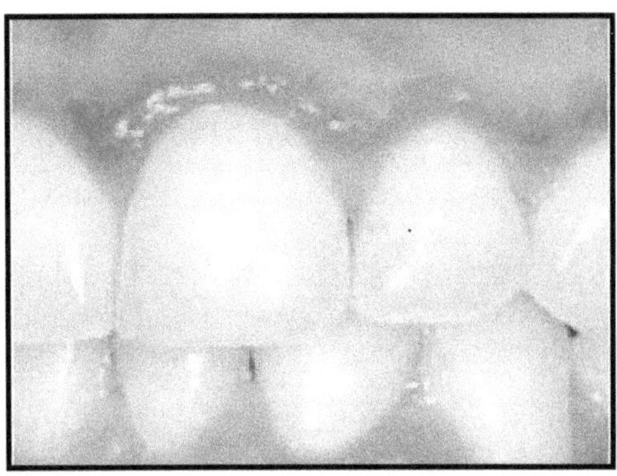

Fig 5. Vitamin C deficiency associated gingival enlargement

3. They bleed spontaneously or on gentle stimulation such as chewing (Stolman 1961).

4. Long standing cases show darkish purple or bluish hue of the tissue.

5. Ulceration may develop and lead to secondary infections.

6. Pseudomembrane formation is common.

7. According to Shaw et al (1978), due to lack of periodontal support, the teeth become mobile. However, Boyle et al (1937) and Waerhaug et al (1958) stated that true loss of attachment and pocket formation do not occur because of the deficiency alone.

Histologic Features[75]

1. Gingival epithelium undergoes thinning. When severe atrophy occurs, blood exudes through breaks in the epithelial layer.

2. The lamina propria shows structural disorganization with poorly formed collagen fibers and thin walled and leaking blood vessels. It has chronic inflammatory cellular infiltration with a superficial acute response. There are scattered areas of hemorrhage with engorged capillaries. Marked diffuse edema, collagen degeneration and scarcity of collagen fibrils or fibroblasts are striking features.[2]

Pathogenesis

Ascorbic acid may play a role in periodontal disease through one or more following suggested mechanisms:[76]

1. Low levels of ascorbic acid influence the metabolism of collagen within the periodontium, affecting the ability of the tissue to regenerate and repair itself.

2. Ascorbic acid deficiency increases the permeability of the oral mucosa to tritiated endotoxins and tritiated inulin and of normal human crevicular epithelium to tritiated dextran (optimal levels of vitamin C would therefore maintain the epithelial barrier to bacterial products).

3. Increasing levels of ascorbic acid enhance both chemotactic and the migratory action of leucocytes without influencing their phagocytic property.

4. An optimal level of ascorbic acid is apparently required to maintain the integrity of the periodontal microvasculature, as well as vascular response to bacterial plaque and wound healing.

5. Depletion of vitamin C may interfere with the ecologic equilibrium of the bacteria in plaque and thus increase its pathogenicity.

Treatment [19]

Ascorbic acid has been found to be beneficial in the treatment of gingivitis when administration was combined with local measures. In addition to administration of ascorbic acid in tablet form, supplementing a diet with fruit juices such as orange, lemon etc also resolves gingivitis (Hanke et al 1933; Thomas 1954, 1962)

Cohen et al (1955) showed that, in the absence of local periodontal treatment, a 500 mg oral of ascorbic acid improved the gingival condition in teenagers after 90 days. According to Cowan et al (1976) daily doses of ascorbic acid (1-3 g) have reduced irregularities in the lamina dura of young adults. Kyhos et al showed that daily 25-75 mg supplement improved periodontal health.

Plasma Cell Gingivitis

Plasma cell gingivitis is a rare inflammatory, non-malignant condition77 of uncertain etiology. It is also referred to as atypical gingivitis or plasma cell gingivostomatitis and often consists of mild marginal gingivitis that extends to the attached gingiva. A localized lesion, referred to as plasma cell granuloma, has also been described.[2]

Etiology

1.   It is a hypersensitivity reaction to some antigen, often spices like red pepper, cardamom.[77]

2.   Flavoring agents such as cinnamonaldehyde and cinnamon in chewing gums and dentifrices were also

shown as etiologic factors in the development of plasma cell gingivitis.[78]

Clinical Features

1.   The patient presents with edematous and inflamed gingiva on the labial aspect of the anterior regions of the maxillary gingiva (Fig 6).[78]

2.   The gingiva appears red, friable, and sometimes granular and bleeds easily.

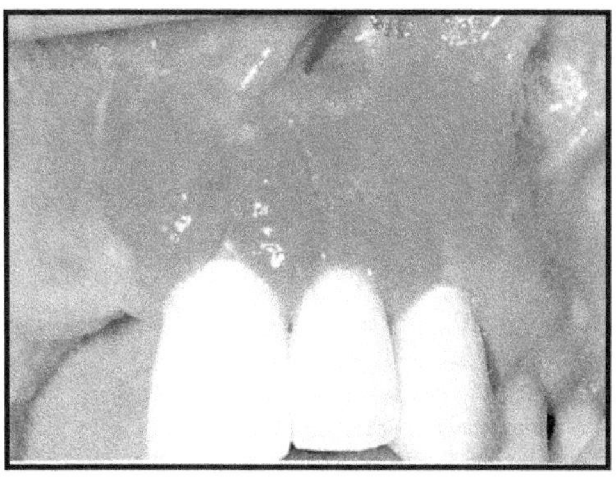

Fig 6. Plasma Cell Gingivitis

3.   It usually does not induce a loss of attachment.[2]

4.   The inflammatory reaction is characterized by intense hyperemic and erythematous changes.

5.   Severe gingival inflammation, discomfort and bleeding and may mimic more serious conditions. An

associated cheilitis and glossitis have also been reported.[77]

6.   In rare instances, marked inflammatory gingival enlargements with predominance of plasma cells can appear associated with aggressive periodontitis.[79]

Histologic Features

1.   Mild epithelial hyperplasia with focal areas of liquefaction, forming microvesicles are seen.[75]

2.   It shows spongiosis[2] and presence of marked leucocytic infiltrate throughout the entire thickness of epithelium.[75]

3.   Ultrastructurally, there are signs of damage in the lower spinous layer and the basal layers.

4.   The underlying connective tissue contains a dense infiltration of plasma cells that extends to the oral epithelium.

5.   There is marked vascular dilatation with severe thinning of epithelium over the connective tissue pegs.

Treatment[19]

In many instances, plasma cell gingivitis resolves on removal of the suspected allergen. Patch test may help to confirm the diagnosis or identify the suspected allergen. In the standard test, the reagents are applied to the skin on the upper back. The skin is then examined after 48 hours for inflammatory reactions. If positive, then the results can be interpreted as a delayed hypersensitivity or local irritant response.

Plasma cell gingivitis is usually a self-limiting condition once the suspected allergen is identified and removed. The patient should be asked to discontinue the use of the suspected allergen like the toothpaste, chewing gum etc. During the period of resolution, the gingival tissues will be sore and hence the patient might be reluctant to carry out regular oral hygiene measures. Administration of topical corticosteroids may facilitate resolution of inflammation.

Non-Specific Conditioned Enlargement (Pyogenic Granuloma)

Pyogenic granuloma is a pedunculated hemorrhagic tumor like gingival enlargement that is considered an exaggerated conditioned response to minor trauma.2 It is of particular significance because of its common intraoral occurrence and because of its sometimes-alarming response.[75]

Poncet and Dor in 1897 first described it as pyogenic granulomal granuloma pyogenicum. Other names were also suggested such as granuloma gravidarum/pregnancy tumour, Crocker and Hartzell's disease, vascular epulis, benign vascular tumour, hemangiomatosis granuloma, epulis teleangiectaticum granulomatosa and lobular capillary hemangioma.[80]

It occurs most frequently on the gingiva and has a strong tendency to recur after simple excision. The name pyogenic granuloma is a misnomer since the condition is not associated with pus and does not represent a granuloma histologically.[75]

Etiology

It was originally believed to be a botryomycotic infection, an infection in horses thought to be transimissible to man. Subsequent work suggested that the lesion was due to infection by either staphylococci or streptococci, partially because it was shown that these microorganisms could produce colonies with fungus-like characteristics.

It is now believed that pyogenic granuloma arises because of some minor trauma to the tissues, which provides pathway for the invasion of nonspecific types of microorganisms. These tissues respond in a characteristic manner to these organisms of low virulence by the overzealous proliferation of a vascular type of connective tissue. The surface of pyogenic granuloma, especially in areas of ulceration, abounds with typical colonies of saprophytic organisms.[75]

Chronic irritation as a causative factor for these lesions may sometimes be hard to identify, but the fact that they are usually located close to the gingival margin suggests that calculus, food materials and overhanging margins of dental restorations are important irritants that should be eliminated when the lesion is excised. These lesions do not occur in mouths that are kept scrupulously free of even minor gingival irritation.[5]

Clinical Features [2,75]

1. The pyogenic granuloma of the oral cavity arises most frequently on the gingiva but may also be found on the lips, tongue and buccal mucosa and occasionally other areas.

2. There is no apparent predilection for any age group.

3. The lesion varies from a discrete spherical, tumor-like pedunculated or sessile mass with a smooth lobulated (Fig 7) or even a warty surface which commonly is ulcerated.

4. It is deep red or reddish purple, depending upon its vascularity.

5. It is soft in consistency and generally is painless in nature.

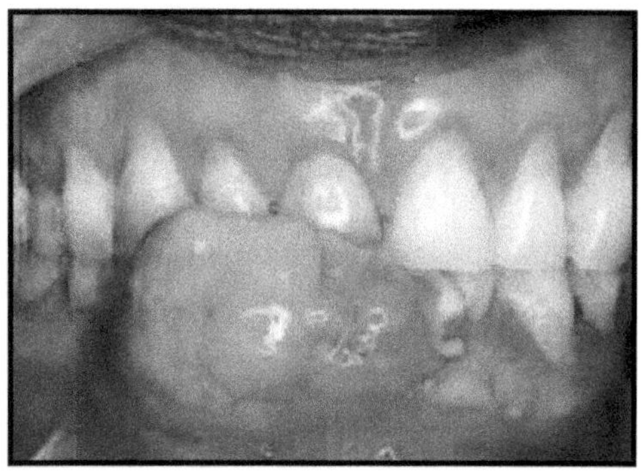

Fig 7. Pyogenic Granuloma in relation to mandibular anterior region

6. It shows a tendency for hemorrhage either spontaneously or upon slight trauma. Some lesions have a brown cast if hemorrhage has occurred into the tissue.

7. Sometimes there is exudation of purulent material, but this is not a characteristic feature despite the suggestive name of this lesion. When such a discharge occurs, it is probably a fistula from an underlying periodontal or periapical abscess.[2]

8. The pyogenic granuloma may develop rapidly, reach full size and then remain static for an indefinite period. The lesions in different cases may vary considerably in size, ranging from a few millimeters to a centimeter or more in diameter.

9. The lesion tends to involute spontaneously to become a fibroepithelial papilloma or persists relatively unchanged for years.

Histologic Features [2,75] *(*Fig.8)

It is like granulation tissue except that it is exuberant and usually well localized.

1. The overlying epithelium, if present, is generally thin and atrophic, but may be hyperplastic.

2. The lesion, if ulcerated, shows a fibrinous exudate of varying thickness over the surface.

3. The most characteristic features are the occurrence of vast numbers of endothelium lined vascular spaces and the extreme proliferation of fibroblasts and budding endothelial cells with minimal collagenous support.

4. The connective tissue stroma is typically delicate, although frequently fasciculi of collagen fibers are noted coursing through the

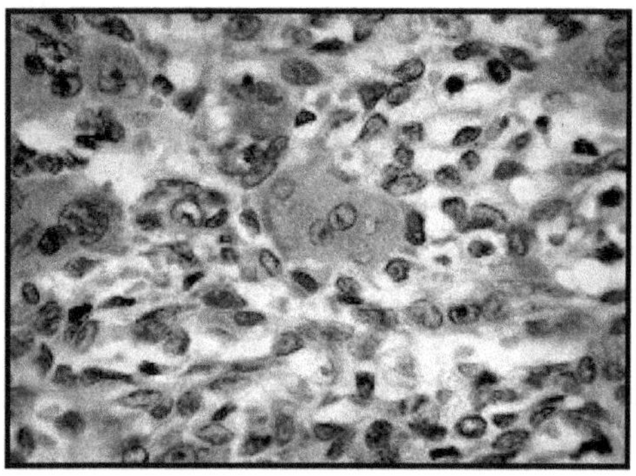

tissue mass.

Fig 8. Histologic section of pyogenic granuloma of the gingiva.

5. There is usually a moderately intense infiltration of polymorphonuclear leucocytes, lymphocytes and plasma cells, but this finding will vary depending upon the presence or absence of ulceration.

6. If the lesion is not excised, there is gradual obliteration of the many capillaries, and it assumes a more fibrous appearance. This maturation of the connective tissue elements is construed as evidence of healing of the lesion.

Radiographic Analysis

Although pyogenic granuloma can be diagnosed clinically with considerable accuracy, radiographic and histopathological investigations aid in confirming the diagnosis and planning the treatment.

Radiographs are advised to rule out bony destruction suggestive of malignancy or to identify a foreign body or sharp restorative margin that would need to be removed with the lesion. Long-standing pyogenic granulomas, like other irritation hyperplasias can show dystrophic calcifications. The radiographic appearances of such calcifications vary from barely perceptible, fine grains of radiopacities to larger, irregular radiopaque particles that rarely exceed 0.5cm in diameter.[80]

Treatment

The existence of these lesions indicates the need for a periodontal consultation and treatment consists of surgical excision of the lesions plus the elimination of irritating local factors. After surgical excision of gingival lesions, curettage of underlying tissue is recommended.

The lesion occasionally recurs because it is not encapsulated, and the surgeon may have difficulty in determining its limits and excising it adequately. While excising it, care must be taken that the adjacent area is free of calculus as that may act as an irritational source and result in re infection. The recurrence rate is about 15%.[73]

Differential Diagnosis

1)   Fibroepithelial polyp or even a typical fibroma.

2)   Pregnancy tumour

3)   Hemangioma

Systemic Diseases Causing Gingival Enlargement

Several systemic diseases may, by different mechanisms, result in gingival enlargement. The diseases most commonly causing gingival enlargement are leukemia, granulomatous diseases like sarcoidosis and Wegener's granulomatosis.

Leukemia-Associated Gingival Enlargement

Leukemia is a heterogeneous group of hematological disorders that arises from a hematopoietic stem cell characterized by disordered differentiation and proliferation of immature white blood cells. This neoplastic proliferation in the marrow is also associated with diminished proliferation of erythrocytes causing anaemia, weakness, fatigue and pallor and platelets causing thrombocytopenia, bleeding, petechiae and bruising. Leukemic cells may also infiltrate spleen, lymph nodes, central nervous system, skin and gingiva.[81]

Due to its high morbidity rate, early diagnosis and appropriate medical therapy is essential. Rapidly forming gingival hyperplasia is usually the first sign of this disease.82 Dentists were responsible for initiating the diagnosis in 25% of patients with acute myelogenous leukemia and 33% of patients with acute myelomonocytic leukemia.[83]

Leukemia is classified as follows[81]

1. According to its clinical behavior

    a. Acute

    b. Chronic

2. According to its histogenetic origin

    a. Lymphocytic

    b. Myelocytic

Clinical Features

Head and neck signs result from leukemic infiltrates or marrow failure. These include cervical lymphadenopathy, oral bleeding, gingival infiltrates, oral infections and oral ulcers.[5]

Oral Manifestations

1. Oral lesions may occur in both acute and chronic forms of all types of leukemia: myeloid, lymphoid and monocytic.[75]

2. True leukemic enlargement occurs commonly in acute leukemia but may also be seen in subacute leukemia. It seldom occurs in chronic leukemia.[2] The leukemic infiltrates in the gingiva are most common in the acute monocytic leukemia and acute myelomonocytic leukemia.[81,82]

3. Leukemic enlargement may be diffuse or marginal, localized or generalized.

4.   It may appear as a diffuse enlargement of the gingival mucosa an oversized extension of the marginal gingiva or a discrete tumor like interproximal mass.

5.   In severe cases, it may almost completely cover the teeth (Fig 9).[75]

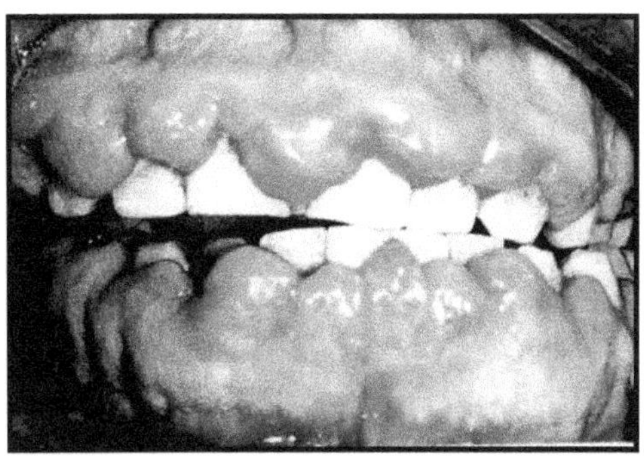

Fig 9. Gingival enlargement in a patient with acute myelocytic leukemia

6.   In leukemic enlargement, the gingiva is generally bluish red and has a shiny surface. The consistency is moderately firm, but there is a tendency toward friability and hemorrhage, occurring either spontaneously or on slight irritation.

7.   Gingival hyperplasia occurs in patients with excellent oral hygiene also, indicating adverse local conditions are not necessary to promote or induce leukemic infiltration of oral tissues.[2]

8.   Poor oral hygiene may predispose the patient to develop infection, bleeding, ulceration and pain.

9.   Acute painful necrotizing ulcerative inflammatory involvement sometimes occurs in the crevice formed at the junction of the enlarged gingiva and the contiguous tooth surfaces.

10.   Patients with leukemia may also have a simple chronic inflammation without the involvement of leukemic cells and may present with the same clinical and microscopic features seen in patients without the disease.

11.   Leukemic infiltrates involving the palate, alveolar bone, and dental pulp also have been reported. Leukemic infiltrates may cause oral signs and symptoms because of the involvement of the fifth and seventh cranial nerves. Disorders of the fifth and seventh cranial nerves also have been reported because of the use of vincristine, a drug commonly used to treat acute lymphocytic leukemia.[5]

Histologic Features

1.   Gingival enlargement in leukemic patients shows various degrees of chronic inflammation with

mature leucocytes and areas of connective tissue infiltrated with a dense mass of immature and proliferating leucocytes, specific nature of which varies with the type of leukemia. Monocytes, when involved, show vesicular nuclei, prominent nucleoli and eosinophilic cytoplasm.[81]

2.   Engorged capillaries, edematous and degenerated connective tissue, epithelium with various degrees of leucocytic infiltration and edema are found.

3.   Isolated surface areas of acute necrotizing inflammation with a pseudomembranous meshwork of fibrin, necrotic epithelial cells, polymorphonuclear neutrophils and bacteria are often seen.[2]

Laboratory Diagnosis

To establish a diagnosis of leukemia, several tests need to do. A complete blood count with differential is the preferred diagnostic test. But a complete and differential blood count would not necessarily identify a lymphoma involving the gingival tissue. Conversely a biopsy helps in appropriate diagnosis of lymphoma showing gingival infiltrates. However, in the earliest phase of gingival involvement, the leukemic infiltrate may be minimal and obscured by a dominant local inflammatory component, thereby masking the neoplastic element.[81]

Differential Diagnosis [81]

The differential diagnosis would include chronic inflammatory gingival enlargement, drug-induced gingival overgrowth, gingival fibrmatoses or neoplastic processes.

Hyperplastic gingivitis secondary to local factors such as periodontal infection or trauma tends to demonstrate erythematous and boggy gingiva localized to a focal area. Drug-induced gingival overgrowth can be caused by anticonvulsants, immunosuppressants and calcium channel blockers. Hereditary gingival fibromatosis presenting generalized gingival enlargement typically occurs before the age of 20 and correlates with tooth eruption and mental retardation.

Treatment[2]

Bleeding and clotting times and platelet count of the patient should be checked and the hematologist consulted before periodontal treatment is instituted.

Firstly, treatment of acute gingival involvement is done. After acute symptoms subside, attention is directed to correction of the gingival enlargement. The rationale is to remove the local irritating factors to control the inflammatory component of the enlargement. The enlargement is treated by scaling and root planing carried out in stages under topical anesthesia. The initial treatment consists of gently removing all loose accumulations with cotton pellets and performing superficial scaling. Treatment is confined to a small area of the mouth to facilitate control of bleeding.

Instructions to the patient should be given for plaque control, which should include daily use of chlorhexidine mouthwashes. Oral hygiene procedures are extremely important in these cases and should be performed by the nurse if necessary. Antibiotics are administered systemically the evening before and for 48 hours after each treatment to reduce the risk of infection. Progressively deeper scaling is carried out at subsequent visits.

Granulomatous Diseases

Granulomatous disorders are a diverse group of diseases that have the presence of non-caseating granulomas in common.[19] Though, Wegener's granulomatosis is a vasculitis, it is characterized by granulomatous lesions and hence discussed under this section.

Sarcoidosis

Sarcoidosis is a multisystem granulomatous disorder of unknown cause.2,84 Evidence implicates improper degradation of antigenic material with the formation of noncaseating granulomatous inflammation. The nature of the antigen is unknown and probably several different antigens may be responsible. The inappropriate defense response may result from prolonged or heavy antigenic exposure, an immune-dysregulation (genetic or secondary to other factors) that prevents an adequate cell-mediated response, a defective regulation of the initial immune reaction or a combination of all three of these factors.84

It has been reported that impairment of chemotaxis is associated with sarcoidosis. Any disorder of neutrophil function will invariably predispose the patient to rapid periodontal breakdown. Thus, in patients with sarcoidosis, the following factors may render them susceptible to periodontal destruction:[19]

1. An increase in B cell activity

2. Secondary infection with A. actinomycetemcomitans

3. An impairment of polymorphonuclear leucocyte chemotaxis.

Etiology[19]

The etiology of sarcoidosis is uncertain. The Third International Conference on sarcoidosis suggested three possible hypotheses:

1. It is due to an unidentified specific agent, and the interaction between this agent and the host is the cause of the immunological peculiarities.

2. It is related to collagenoses or to reticuloses, in which immunological changes are prominent.

3. It occurs only in individuals who have a pre-existing immunological peculiarity, and develop a reaction to an agent, or one of several agents, which may or may not be known already as causing some well-known disease (eg. tuberculosis).

Clinical Features

Although any organ may be affected, the lungs, lymph nodes, skin, eyes and salivary glands are the predominant sites.[2,5,84] Clinically evident oral manifestations in sarcoidosis are uncommon.

1. It starts in second or third decade, predominantly affecting blacks.[2,84]

2. The most frequently affected intraoral soft tissue site is the buccal mucosa, followed by the gingiva, lips, floor of mouth, tongue and palate.

3. The mucosal lesions may be normal in color, brownish- red, violaceous, or hyperkeratotic.

4. Sarcoidosis involving the gingiva shows a red, smooth, painless enlargement (Fig 10).

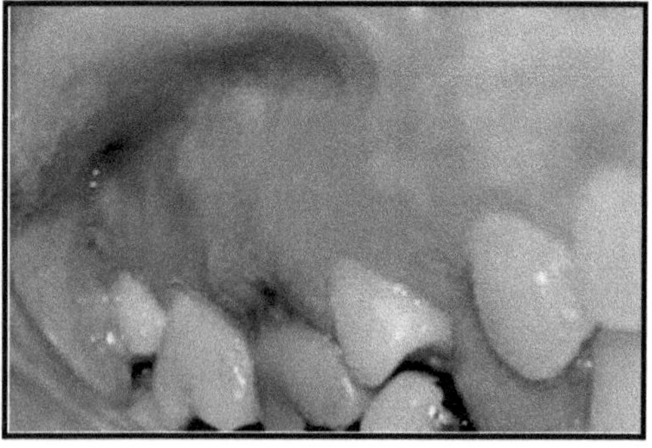

Fig 10. Initial clinical presentation of gingival sarcoidosis.

5. It may also appear as a submucosal mass, an isolated papule, or an area of granularity.[84]

6. Severe and rapid periodontal destruction has been reported as an oral complication of sarcoidosis.

Histologic Features

Sarcoid granulomas consist of discrete, non-caseating whorls of epithelioid cells and multi nucleated foreign body type giant cells with peripheral mononuclear cells. The granuloma may contain inclusion bodies referred to as the Schaumann or conchoids body the asteroid body, and microcentrosomes.[19]

Treatment

Surgical excision of the gingival overgrowth should be done. However, unless the underlying systemic disease is not treated or kept under control, recurrence will occur.[19]

Wegener's Granulomatosis

Wegener's granulomatosis is a rare disease characterized by acute granulomatous necrotizing lesions of the respiratory tract, including nasal and oral defects. Renal lesions also develop, and acute necrotizing vasculitis affects the blood vessels. It was first described in 1936 by Friedrich Wegener.[19,85]

A pathological triad[19] has been described for this condition consisting of:

1. Necrotizing granulomas in the nose, paranasal sinuses, and lungs

2. Vasculitis of small arteries and veins

3. Glomerulitis is characterized by necrosis of loops of the glomerular capillary tufts, capsular adhesion and granulomatous lesions.

Etiology

The etiology is obscure. It may be an immunological disorder as it responds to immunosuppressive therapy.

Clinical Features

1.   The initial manifestations of Wegener's granulomatosis may involve the orofacial region and include oral mucosal ulceration, gingival enlargement, abnormal tooth mobility, exfoliation of teeth and delayed healing response.[2]

2.   Oral involvement appears in 10% to 62% of patients with Wegener's granulomatosis particularly affecting the tongue and the gingiva.[86]

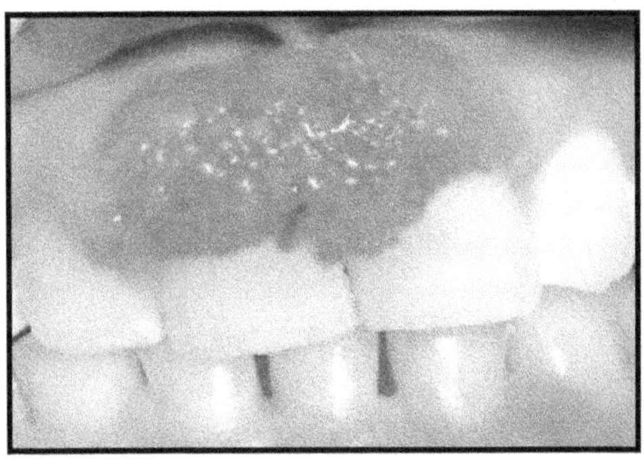

Fig 11. – Strawberry- like gingival tumour in Wegener's granulomatosis.

3.   The clinical patterns observed at the gingiva may include the presence of diffuse gingivitis, diffuse inflammatory overgrowth affecting the free and attached gingiva or the presence of a gingival enlargement showing a typical granular surface. The latter has been

termed ''strawberry gingiva'. This hyperplastic diffuse gingivitis has been considered a pathognomonic sign in cases of Wegener's granulomatosis (Fig 11).

4.   The granulomatous papillary enlargement is reddish purple and bleeds easily on stimulation.[2]

Histologic Features[19] (Fig 12)

1.   It shows non-specific, chronic histiocytic inflammation.

2.   The overlying epithelium invariably shows pseudoepitheliomatous hyperplasia and eosinophilia.

3.   Microabscesses, multinucleated giant cells, focal necrosis, fibrinoid degeneration and vasculitis are seen in some cases.

4.   Gingival vascular changes like swelling and necrosis of the endothelial cells, along with eosinophilic granulocytes and plasma cells around the capillary wall may be seen.

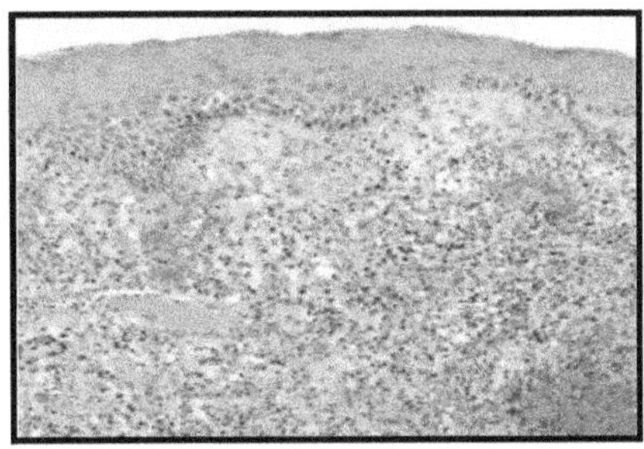

Fig 12. Histologic section of Wegener's granulomatosis of the gingiva.

Treatment

Institution of systemic drug therapy like prednisolone and cyclophosphamide bring about improvement in the gingival conditions. A case report by Raustia et al 1985 showed that attention to plaque control had little effect on the gingival appearance.

Differential Diagnosis

1.   Malignant tumors. However, the margins of the lesion are generally more diffuse and infiltrative than those seen in lesions in Wegener's granulomatosis.

2.   Other disorders including leukemia, pregnancy gingivitis, drug-induced gingival overgrowth and others could be excluded by the patient's medical and dental history, physical examination and laboratory analyses.

6. Idiopathic Gingival Enlargement

Idiopathic gingival enlargement is a rare condition of unknown etiology. It is designated by terms such as fibromatosis gingivae, gingivomatosis, hereditary gingival fibromatosis, idiopathic fibromatosis, familial elephantiasis, and diffuse fibroma.[2]

Hereditary gingival fibromatosis (HGF) is an inherited condition in which the gingival tissue enlarges spontaneously and progressively. It is a rare autosomal dominant disease occurring in infancy. Gross in 1856 reported the first case.[87]

Clinical features (Fig. 1)

Gingiva is firm, leathery in consistency and of normal color with a typical minutely pebbled surface.

It is asymptomatic as well as non-hemorrhagic. The attached gingiva as well as the interdental papilla, and the gingival margin are affected.[2]

It is heterogeneous condition with enlargement being generalized or localized to characteristically to the labial gingiva around the mandibular molars and maxillary tuberosities. It usually commences with eruption of the permanent dentition, however, can develop with deciduous dentition eruption. The condition is rarely there at birth and usually non-detectable in adults. The enlargement tends to recede with tooth loss.[87]

Teeth are practically entirely covered in severe cases with the enlargement projecting into the vestibule. The bulbous gingival enlargement makes the jaw look distorted. The enlargement is usually superimposed with secondary inflammatory changes at the gingival margin.

The gingival enlargement does not directly affect the alveolar bone, however the accumulation of bacterial plaque due to gingival swelling lead to halitosis, periodontitis, and alveolar bone resorption.

The condition results in functional and esthetic issues like teeth malpositioning, diastemas, delayed eruption, continued retention of primary dentition, prominent lips, open and cross bites, and open lip posture.

The enlargement in few instances may be associated with hypertrichosis and retardation of physical development.[2]

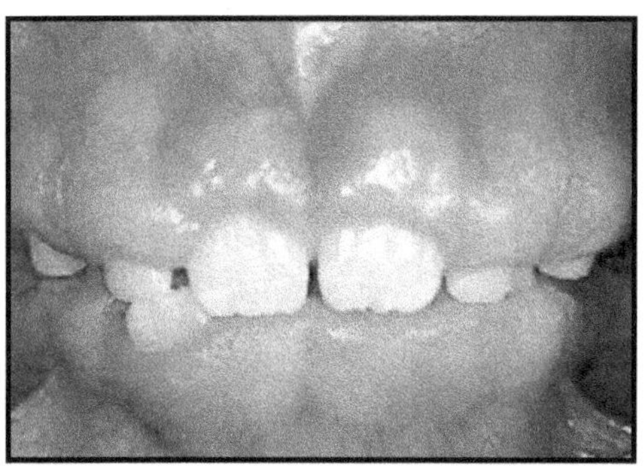

Fig 1– Hereditary gingival fibromatosis.

There is an increase in the number of bundles of collagen fibers, accompanying a few fibroblasts (Fig 2). There are types of fibroblasts present, one associated with dense collagen bundles containing little cytoplasm, considered inactive and the active ones with abundant rough and smoot endoplasmic reticulum, numerous mitochondria, a well-developed Golgi apparatus. Subepithelial connective tissue frequently has mild chronic inflammatory infiltrates.

There are no proliferating fibroblasts in the connective tissue as evaluated by expression of the markers proliferating cellular nuclear antigen (PCNA) and pKi-67.

The epithelium is well-structured with thin and elongated papillae inserted in fibrous connective tissue. Some zones of epithelial atrophy may be seen. Areas with intense chronic inflammation showed prominent papillae and epithelial hyperplasia and only long and deep epithelial papillae were seen in areas without inflammation Raeste et al. (1978).

Some rare findings, like amyloid deposits, islands of odontogenic epithelium small, calcified particles, osseous metaplasia, and ulceration of the covering mucosa are also found.

Pallavi Sharma, Dwiti Thanawala,
Alankrita Chaudhary, Himani Sharma

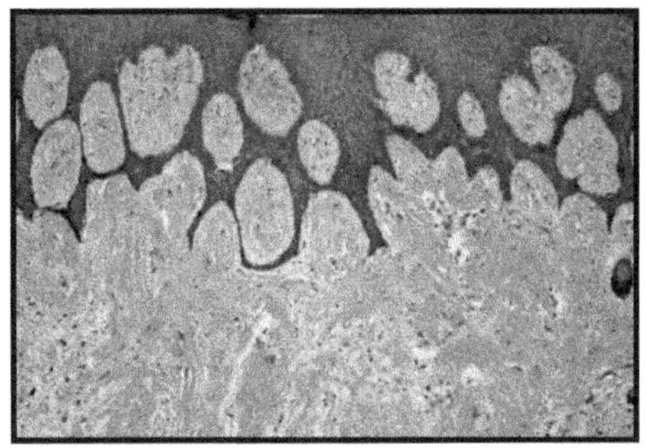

Fig 2– Histologic section of hereditary gingival fibromatosis.

The histologic features of HGF are non-specific and the definitive diagnosis requires correlation with clinical findings and family history.

Syndromes associated with hereditary gingival fibromatosis

Hereditary gingival fibromatosis is frequently an isolated disorder, but in few cases, it is associated with other changes suggestive of a syndrome (Table 1). The syndromic characteristic most seen in association with HGF is hypertrichosis, which is occasionally associated with mental retardation.

Syndrome	Inheritance	Features Apart From Gingival Fibromatosis
Gingival fibromatosis with hypertrichosis	AD	Hypertrichosis, mental retardation
Zimmermann-Laband	AD	Ear and nose defects, dysplastic nails, terminal phalanges hypoplastic, joint hyperextensibility, and hepatosplenomegaly
Murray-Puretic-Drescher (juvenile hyaline fibromatosis)	AR	Multiple hyaline fibromas, osteolysis of terminal phalanges, recurrent infections, stunted growth, and premature death
Rutherfurd	AD	Corneal opacities and retarded tooth eruption
Gingival fibromatosis with distinctive facies	AR	Macrocephaly, hypertelorism, bushy eyebrows with synophrys, downslanted palpebral fissures, flat nasal bridge, hypoplastic nares, Cupid's bow mouth, and highly arched palate
Ramon	AR	Cherubism, hypertrichosis, mental deficiency, epilepsy, stunted growth, juvenile rheumatoid arthritis, and ocular abnormalities
Cross	AR	Microphthalmia, mental retardation, athetosis, and hypopigmentation
Jones	AD	Progressive deafness
Prune-belly	Unclear	Absence of abdominal muscles, abnormalities of urinary tract, cryptorchidism, and facial dimorphism

Table 1. Syndromes associated with HGF.

(AD: Autosomal dominant, AR: Autosomal recessive)

Genetic findings in hereditary gingival fibromatosis

Three distinct loci have been linked with the isolated form of HGF: two mappings to chromosome 2

(GINGF on 2p21-22 and GINGF3 on 2p22.3-p23.3), which do not overlap, and one to chromosome 5 (GINGF2 on 5q13-q22). Of these, SOS1 (son of sevenless one) gene underlying the GINGF locus has been discovered. The SOS1 mutation was studied in a large multigenerational Brazilian family segregating HGF as a highly penetrant autosomal dominant gene.[88]

Pathogenesis

Fibroblasts from HGF proliferate quicker than normal gingiva as confirmed by studies.[89]

Elevated levels of fatty acid synthase (FAS) and androgen receptor are produced by highly proliferative HGF cells, indicating a role for the androgen-driven fatty acid biosynthesis in fibroblast proliferation in HGF. There seems to be a role of sex hormones on gingival enlargement as indicated by testosterone induced proliferation and production of interleukin-6 (IL-6) by HGF fibroblasts.

Patients with HGF demonstrated both increase and decrease in collagen synthesis, with 30% to 50% increase in collagen production as compared to normal gingival fibroblasts [89,90] The major type produced by

HGF is Type I collagen along with increased production of heat shock protein 47 (Hsp47), a precise molecular chaperone for type I collagen that binds to it. Hsp47 may play a key role in the posttranslational processing of the overproduced type I procollagen chains, causing buildup of collagen in HGF gingiva.

Diminished degradation of extracellular matrix as well as enhanced synthesis of extracellular matrix components, such as glycosaminoglycans and fibronectin are seen in HGF leading to gingival enlargement in HGF (Fig. 3).[87,89]

Collagen degradation can be caused by either degradation by matrix metalloproteinases (MMP) or fibroblast phagocytosis and impaired expression and activity of MMP-1 and MMP-2 has been explained in HGF cells. [87,90] Thus, the decrease of the degradative capacity of HGF cells may lead to enhanced collagen content.

Cytokines and growth factors control the proliferation and metabolism of the connective tissue. Unusually higher levels of transforming growth factor beta 1 (TGF-β1), TGF- β2 and TGF- β3 and IL-6 are observed in gingival enlargement due to HGF. [87] This attributed to the promotion of increased levels of type I collagen and Hsp47 and a reduction in MMP-1 and MMP-2 expression by normal gingival fibroblasts by adding TGF-β1 and IL-6.[90]

Furthermore, TGF-β1 enhances fibroblast proliferation as well leads to the induction of myofibroblast trans-differentiation via connective tissue growth factor (CTGF) pathway leading to excessive accumulation of the extracellular matrix. Myofibroblasts are responsible for contraction of wounds, restoration of the connective tissue during wound healing, as well as excessive collagen accumulation.[87]

Thus, HGF is heterogeneous in its clinical and genetic features as well as in the biologic characteristics of cultured cells.

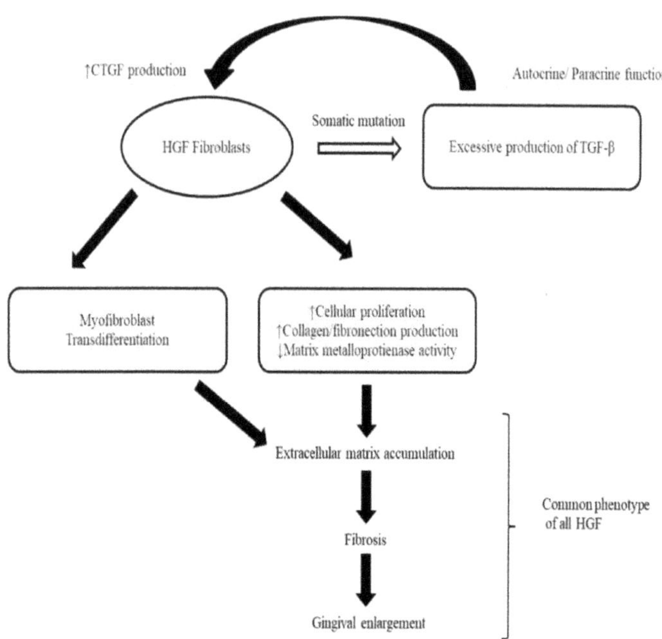

Fig. 3. A model for the pathogenesis of HGF. Somatic mutations result in gingival fibroblasts with elevated synthesis of TGF- β, which, in an autocrine and paracrine fashion, promotes cellular proliferation, abnormally high collagen and fibronectin production and reduces the synthesis and activity of matrix-metalloproteinases.

Additionally, TGF- β 1 may induce fibroblast trans-differentiation into myofibroblasts, all the actions of TGF- β result in a dysregulation of the connective tissue homeostasis, leading to the accumulation of extracellular matrix, which clinically culminates in gingival enlargement.

Treatment[87]

With respect to the period in which the treatment must be attempted, several authors believe the most appropriate time is after eruption of the permanent dentition as it decreases the risk of recurrence. However, in certain cases, it may lead to prolonged retention of the primary dentition and delayed eruption of the permanent teeth, esthetic as well as psychological complications, teeth malpositioning and difficulties in mastication and phonation.

Treatment varies according to the severity of enlargement. With minimal enlargement, thorough scaling and root planing and good oral hygiene maintenance at home is usually sufficient whereas surgical excision is required for overgrown gingival tissues.

Various techniques including internal or external bevel gingivectomy along with gingivoplasty, electrocautery and carbon dioxide laser, or apically positioned flap have been used for excision of the gingiva. Though unpredictable, recurrence is usually noticed early due to inadequate oral hygiene maintenance.

Pallavi Sharma, Dwiti Thanawala,
Alankrita Chaudhary, Himani Sharma

7. Neoplasms

Neoplasms form comparatively lesser proportion of gingival enlargements and make up only a small percentage of the total number of oral neoplasms.

Benign tumors of the gingiva

Epulis is a generic clinical term used to refer to all discrete tumors and tumor-like masses of the gingiva. Most of the lesions referred to as epulis are inflammatory.[2]

Fibromas

Fibromas are the most widespread benign soft tissue neoplasms of oral cavity. It is most seen on the gingiva, buccal mucosa, tongue, lips, and palate.[75] fibromas of the gingiva usually arise from either gingival connective tissue or periodontal ligament.

Clinical features

1. It can occur at any age, but most seen in the third, fourth and fifth decades.[75]

2. It occurs as an elevated lesion of normal color (Fig 1). It has a smooth surface and usually a sessile and sometimes a pedunculated base.[75]

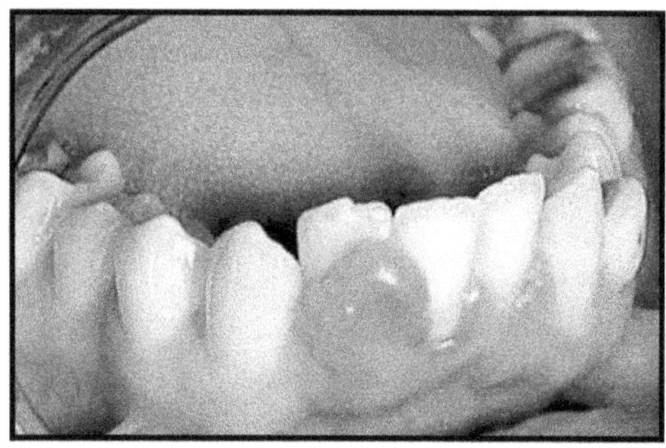

Fig 1– Fibroma of the gingiva in relation to 41, 42.

3. It is nearly always a well-defined, vascular, and slow growing spherical tumor.

4. The consistency may be firm, resilient, and nodular or soft and spongy.

5. It may occasionally become inflamed and irritated displaying superficial ulceration.

6. The peripheral ossifying fibroma, occurring solely on the gingiva, is relatively common, found most often in the maxillary anterior region, and rarely in the mandibular area.[93]

7. Rarely a peripheral ossifying fibroma lesion may be accompanied by tooth migration, and radiographic signs of radiolucency suggestive of bone destruction and radiopacity suggestive of calcifications. [93,94]

Histologic features

Fibromas are comprised of well-formed collagen fiber bundles with scattered fibrocytes and a varying vascularity. Multi-nucleated fibroblasts are found in giant cell fibroma. Keratinized or parakeratotic stratified squamous epithelium with ulcerations in 20 percent cases is seen in peripheral ossifying fibroma. Highly cellular fibrous tissue with regions of calcifications (cementum like material, bone, or dystrophic calcifications) are seen in the connective tissue.[75]

Treatment

The treatment of choice is complete excision including the involved periosteum and periodontal ligament. If the excision is performed without simultaneous periodontal therapy, there may be chances recurrence in <10% cases.[93]

Differential diagnosis[75]

The differential diagnosis of gingival fibroma includes common localized gingival lesions, e.g., fibrous hyperplasia, pyogenic granuloma, peripheral giant cell granuloma and rare ones, e.g. Peripheral odontogenic fibroma.

Since clinical characteristics of the above-mentioned lesions do not offer adequate characteristic features for differentiation from each other, histopathological analysis turns into a crucial diagnostic tool.

Traumatic neuroma

The traumatic neuroma occurs as a reaction to trauma or peripheral nerve transection representing a futile effort at repairing the nerve.[95] the proliferating proximal nerve fibers are unsuccessful in fusing with the distal segment because of the intervening scar tissue.

Clinical features[95]

1. A typical clinical presentation is that of a tender nodule in the mental foramen, on the edentulous mandibular mucosa.

2. Another common location is in the posterior part of the mandible after the impacted third molar extraction. Lower lip and tongue are the other frequent sites of occurrence.

Histologic features

It is comprised of an irregularly proliferating mature nerve bundles in a dense or loosely arranged fibrous stroma.

Treatment

Treatment involves surgical excision of the enlarged mass as well as a small part of the involved nerve segment. Recurrence is not common.

Neurofibroma

The neurofibroma is a benign tumor composed of perineural fibroblasts, schwann cells, and neural cells or axons. It can either occur as a solitary lesion or as multiple lesions associated with neurofibromatosis (von recklinghausen's disease).[75,95]

Clinical features

1. Solitary neurofibromas characteristically present as slow growing, non-ulcerated, usually asymptomatic

soft tissue nodules, of the color same as that of surrounding mucosa or skin, may occur intraorally or on the skin. (Fig. 2).

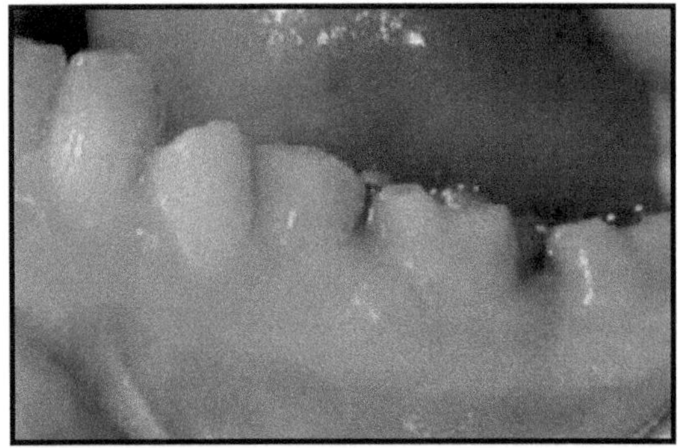

Fig 2– Neurofibroma of the gingiva in relation to 35, 36.

2. The most common oral sites are the tongue and buccal mucosa and rarely gingiva.
3. It occurs most frequently in the second and third decades of life but may occur at any age.

Histologic features

1. Typically non-encapsulated, the lesions may display a cellular proliferation of small spindle cells, many of which demonstrate wavy nuclei intermingled with neuritis in an irregular

pattern with intertwining connective tissue fibrils.[75, 95]

2. Several mast cells are usually scattered throughout the lesion.

3. Melanocytes may sometimes be found.

Treatment

The treatment of choice is conservative surgical excision for solitary neurofibroma. Recurrence is unusual.

Papilloma

The papilloma is a benign neoplasm which is common in occurrence and originates form the surface epithelium.[75] the human papillomavirus (HPV) is associated with it, the most common subtypes being hpv-6 and hpv-11[.2]

Clinical features

1. An exophytic lesion with several small finger-like projections.

2. Commonly occurs as a well-circumscribed pedunculated tumor, occasionally it may be sessile.

3. Intraorally most found on the tongue, lips, buccal mucosa, gingiva, and palate.

4. This lesion is seen to occur in all age groups.75

5. Gingival papillomas may either be seen as a wartlike or cauliflower-like solitary lesion, (Fig. 3) or it may be discrete and small or broad, hard elevations with minutely irregular surfaces.[2]

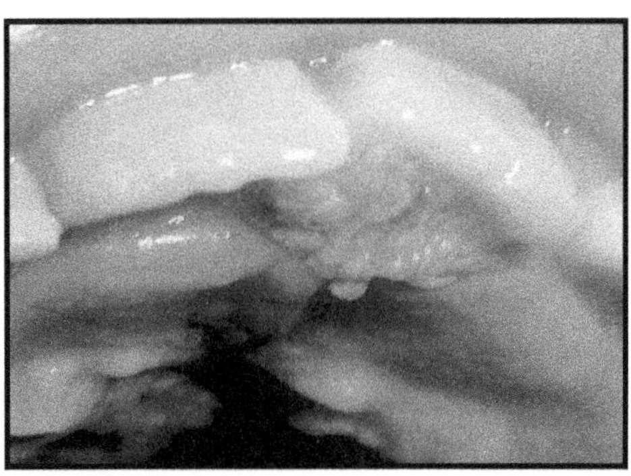

Fig. 3– Papilloma in relation to 11, 12

6. Usually, they are only few millimeters in diameter, sometimes may grow up to several centimeters.

Histologic features[2,75]

It consists of several thin and long finger-like projections which extend from the mucosal surface.

These projections contain thin, central connective tissue core supporting the blood vessels with an outer continuous layer of stratified squamous epithelium. The essential feature is papillary proliferation of the spinous cells. The connective tissue is only present in the supportive stroma and is not a part of the neoplastic element. Mitotic activity in the epithelial cells is sometimes disturbingly prevalent. Chronic inflammatory cells may be inconsistently present in the connective tissue.

Treatment

Complete surgical excision including the of the base of mucosa where the pedicle inserts is recommended. Recurrence is rare if the tumor is excised completely. Malignant degermation is quite unusual.[75]

Peripheral giant cell granuloma

Peripheral giant cell granuloma is an uncommon proliferative reaction of the tissues to injury. The usual cause of trauma is tooth extraction, other significant causes being persistent chronic infection or irritation from dentures. The granuloma either originates from mucoperiosteum or the periodontal ligamen.[75]

historically, peripheral giant cell granulomas were referred to as peripheral reparative giant cell tumors. The nomenclature was changes after the understanding that these lesions were responses to local injury and not neoplasms and their reparative nature has not been established.[2]

Clinical features[2,75]

1. Frequency of occurrence is twice in females when compared to males

2. Occurs more commonly in the mandible

3. Occurs on gingiva or alveolar process, usually anterior to the molars

4. The lesion may be pedunculated or sessile usually arising from deeper in the tissues

5. It arises interdentally or from the gingival margin, with predilection for the labial surface.

6. Lesion may be spongy or firm

7. The color differs from pink to deep red or purplish blue.

8. The lesion differs widely in size, typically between 0.5 - 1.5 cm in diameter.

9. Lesions are painless except if the margins are ulcerated.

10. They vary in appearance from smooth, regularly outlined masses to multilobulated irregularly shaped protuberances with indentations on the surface.

11. Sometimes it may be locally invasive leading to destruction of the underlying bone.

Histologic features[2,75]

1. It comprises of a non-encapsulated mass of tissue composed of delicate reticular and fibrillar connective tissue stroma containing large number of ovoid or spindle-shaped young connective tissue cells and multinucleated giant cells (Fig. 4).

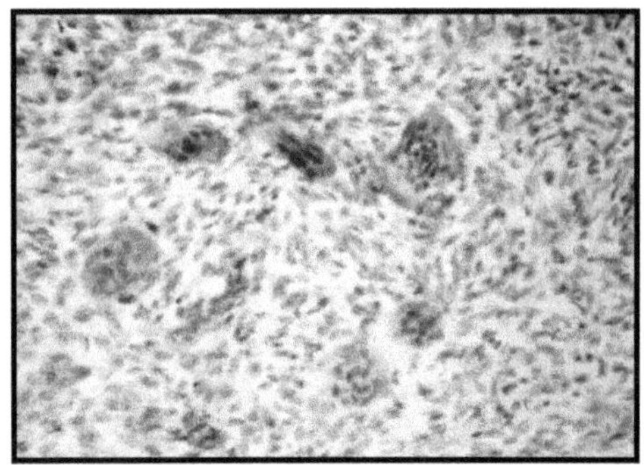

Fig. 4– Histologic section of peripheral giant cell granuloma showing giant cells

2. Numerous capillaries are present, especially around the periphery of the lesion, and the giant cells occasionally may be found within the lumina of these vessels.

3. Foci of hemorrhage with emancipation of hemosiderin pigment and its consequent ingestion by mononuclear phagocytes, along with inflammatory cell infiltration are distinguishing features of the lesion.

4. Areas of chronic inflammation are scattered throughout the lesion with acute involvement occurring at the surface.

5. Spicules of newly formed osteoid or bone are often found scattered throughout the vascular and cellular fibrous lesion.

6. The epithelium is typically hyperplastic with ulceration occurring at the base.

Radiographic features

Evidence of involvement of the underlying bone may or may not be evident from the intraoral radiographs. In edentulous regions, the peripheral giant cell granuloma typically exhibits erosion of the bone superficially with peripheral "cuffing" of the bone. Superficial destruction of the alveolar margin or the crest of the interdental bone is noticed in dentulous regions.[75]

Treatment[2,75]

Surgical excision of the lesion, including the base of the lesion, is the preferred treatment. If only superficial excision is carried out, recurrence is possible. Complete removal leads to uneventful recovery.

Central giant cell granuloma

These lesions occur within the jaws and create central cavitation and sometimes produce a distortion of the jaw that makes the gingiva seem enlarged (Fig. 5).

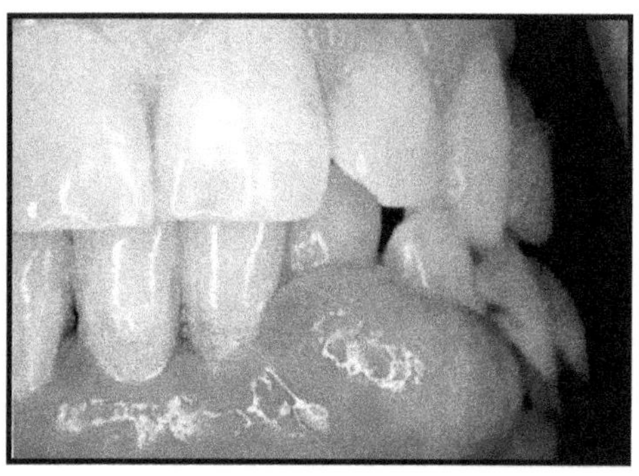

Fig. 5– Central giant cell granuloma in relation to 31, 32 and 33.

Leukoplakia

The World health organization defined leukoplakia as a white patch or plaque that does not rub off and cannot be diagnosed as any other disease. It is precisely a clinical term.[95]

Etiology

Although the etiology of leukoplakia remains unclear, it is usually correlated with the use of tobacco (smoke or smokeless). Various chemical constituents of tobacco and its combustion end products, such as tobacco tars and resins, are aggravating substances which can cause leukoplakic alterations of the oral mucosa.[95]

Other probable factors are candida albicans, hpv-16 and hpv-18, alcohol, vitamin deficiency, trauma, or chronic irritation due to ill-fitting dentures, cheek biting, sharp broken teeth, ultraviolet radiation etc. [75, 95]

Clinical features

1. Leukoplakia is most seen in adults over 40 years of age, with a significant male predilection.
2. Buccal mucosa and commissures are most involved, followed in the descending order by the alveolar mucosa, tongue, lip, hard and soft palate, floor of the mouth and gingiva.[75]
3. Leukoplakia of the gingiva can be seen as grayish white, flattened, scaly lesion or a thick, irregularly-shaped keratinous plaque (Fig. 6).

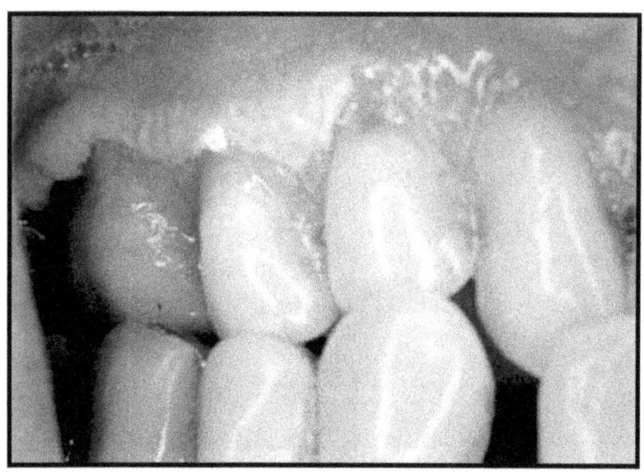

Fig. 6– Leukoplakia of the gingiva.

Histologic features

1. It exhibits hyperkeratosis and acanthosis (Fig. 7).

2. Premalignant and malignant cases have a variable degree of atypical epithelial changes that may be mild, moderate, or severe, depending on the extent of the involvement of the epithelial layers.[2]

3. When dysplastic changes involve all the layers, it is diagnosed as carcinoma in situ, and this may become invasive carcinoma when the basement membrane is breached. [95]

4. Inflammatory involvement of the underlying connective tissue is a commonly associated finding.

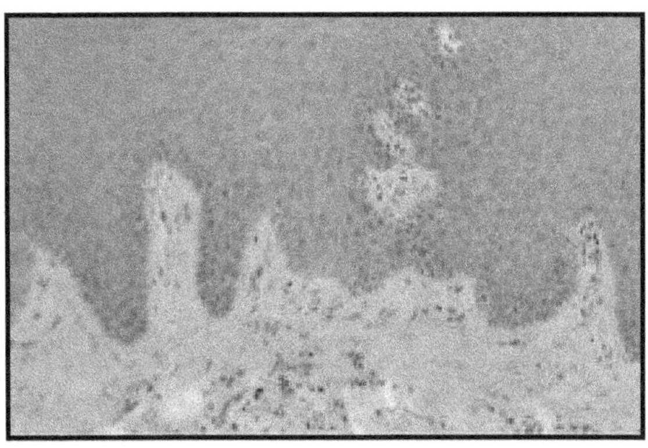

Fig. 7– Histologic section of leucoplakia of the gingiva.

About 80% of leukoplakias are benign, about 20% are malignant or premalignant and only 3% are invasive carcinomas. To come to the correct diagnosis and establish appropriate therapy, it is necessary to take biopsy of all leukoplakias, from the most suspicious region.[95]

Treatment

There exist several opinions regarding treatment of leukoplakia, it is usually considered that lesions with moderate or severe epithelial dysplasia or carcinoma in situ must be entirely removed either by surgical excision, electrosurgery, laser therapy, or cryosurgery. The use of topical and/or systemic vitamin a analogue in the treatment of leukoplakia have demonstrated inconsistent results.[96] to track recurrences, long-term follow-up is necessary.[95]

Gingival cyst

The gingival cyst is an unusual cyst of the gingival soft tissue. It can occur in either free or attached gingiva. The cysts grow from odontogenic epithelium or from surface or sulcular epithelium traumatically implanted in the region. Although gingival cysts of microscopic dimensions are common, they occasionally grow to a clinically considerable size.

Clinical features[2,75]

1. They appear as localized lesions that may involve the free and/or the attached gingiva.

2. Usually occurs in the mandibular canine - premolar regions, with a predilection for lingual surface.

3. Present as small, well-circumscribed, painless swelling of the gingiva.

4. The same color is usually the same as the adjacent mucosa and rarely measures more than 1 cm in diameter.

5. Painless lesions but if they expand it may lead to the erosion of the surface of the alveolar bone.

Histologic features

The cyst cavity is covered by a thin stratified squamous epithelium, with or without localized areas of thickening. The thickness may vary from one flattened cell to numerous cells. Sometimes, the following types of epithelia may be seen, non-keratinized or keratinized stratified squamous epithelium, or parakeratinized epithelium with palisading basal cells.[2]

Glycogen rich clear cells may be present, particularly in the plaques or focal thickenings of the lining. The cyst may or may not exhibit an inflammatory response as it remains free in the connective tissue of the gingiva.[75]

Differential diagnosis[95]

Lateral periodontal cyst – it occurs within the alveolar bone, adjacent to the root and is developmental in origin. Other rare benign tumors including nevus, hemangioma, myoblastoma, mucus-secreting cysts (mucoceles) and ameloblastoma[2]

Malignant tumors of the gingiva

Oral cancer constitutes less than 3% of all malignant tumors in the body. It is however the 6th most common cancer in males and the 12th in females. Gingiva is not a common site of oral malignancy accounting for only 6% of oral cancers.

Squamous cell carcinoma

Squamous cell carcinoma is the most frequent malignant tumor of the gingiva accounting for more than 90% of all oral cancers.

Etiology

The etiology of carcinoma of the gingiva is not very well-defined or specific and is reliant on over one causative factor. The most plausible cofactors implicated in the causation of squamous cell carcinoma, are use of tobacco, alcohol, human papilloma viruses, chronic iron deficiency anemia, immunosuppression and oncogene and tumor suppressor gene dysregulation.95 chronic irritation because of the presence of calculus and microorganisms could also contribute to the incidence of carcinoma of the gingiva. Occasionally, it occurs after extraction of teeth.[75]

Clinical features

1. Gingival squamous cell carcinomas are seen in both maxilla and mandible with a slight a predilection for mandibular gingiva.[75, 95]

2. Gingival squamous cell carcinoma occurs more frequently in females than males.[95]

3. It is goes unnoticed without symptoms until complicated by superimposed inflammatory changes that causes pain.

4. Leukoplakic or erythron-leukoplakic lesion with a pebbly surface is the characteristic presentation for gingival squamous cell carcinoma.

5. Sometimes it may present as an exophytic irregular outgrowth, or ulcerative, flat, erosive lesions (Fig. 8).

6. Sometimes, gingival squamous cell carcinomas may establish as a rapidly growing lesion originating from a current extraction site most likely occurring due to the downgrowth of tumor along the periodontal ligament and its ensuing proliferation following extraction.

7. They are locally invasive, affecting the underlying bone and periodontal ligament of adjacent teeth and the adjoining mucosa. In the maxilla, maxillary sinuses or the tonsillar pillars may be affected. In the mandible, it commonly extends into the floor of the mouth or laterally into the cheek.[75]

8. Metastasis is typically restricted to the area above the clavicle; however, more extensive

involvement may include the lung, liver or bone.

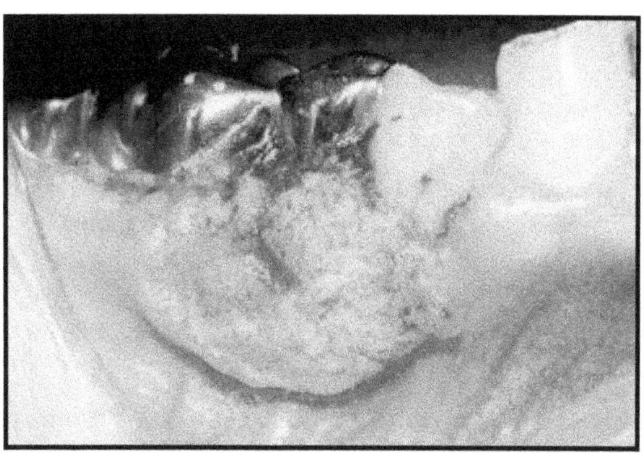

Fig. 8– Squamous cell carcinoma of the gingiva.

Histologic features

Microscopically, most gingival squamous cell carcinomas are moderately or well-differentiated tumors.[95] underlying connective tissue is invaded by islands of clearly identifiable squamous cells. Mitoses individual cell keratinization and keratin pearl formation, nuclear hyperchromatism and pleomorphism, may be detected.

Differential diagnosis

Gingival squamous cell carcinoma may mimic inflammatory or reactive conditions affecting the gingiva and periodontium such as gingivitis, periodontitis, pyogenic granuloma, dental infection like endo-periodontic lesion, neoplasms like leukoplakia and erythroplakia.[97]

Treatment

Surgical excision is the preferred treatment. Wide-ranging local excision involving the underlying bone is most often employed. Marginal mandibulectomy appears to be effective in mandibular lesions with no or minimal bone invasion. If the primary tumor is superficial and small, supra-omohyoid dissection of the ipsilateral neck is suggested even in the presence of clinically negative nodes.

Post-operative radiotherapy is used for patients with occult cervical metastases, positive surgical margins, or advanced stage disease. The general 5-year survival rate for gingival squamous cell carcinoma is around 54%.[95]

Malignant melanoma

Melanoma is a malignant melanocytic neoplasm most observed on the skin, however, may arise at any region where melanocytes are present. Melanoma arising in the mucous membranes of the head and neck comprises approximately 2% of all melanomas. [95]

Etiology

The etiology of oral melanoma is still unknown.[95]

Clinical features (Fig. 9)

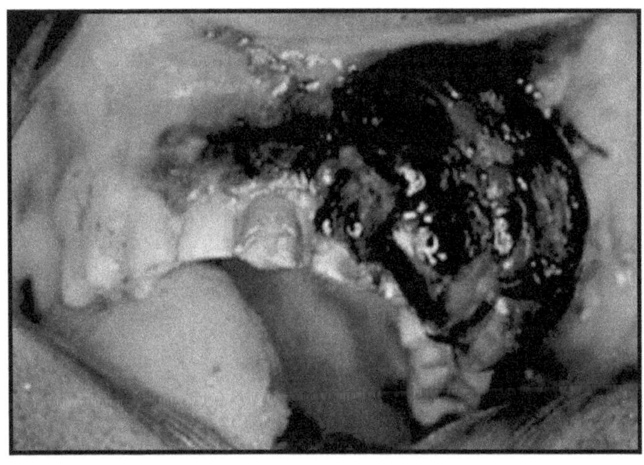

Fig. 9– Malignant melanoma of the gingiva.

Malignant melanoma is a rare oral tumor usually occurring in the hard palate and maxillary gingiva, arising from the melanoblasts of gingiva, cheek, or palate.

1. They may occur as multiple or synchronous lesions.

2. Oral melanomas are typically brown or black lesions, 1 to 4 cm in size, which may be nodular or flat with a rapid rate of growth. With time lesions tend to become darker and larger with irregular borders and ultimately develop ulceration and bleeding[2,95]

3. Oral melanomas are characterized by early metastasis, infiltrating the underlying bone. Cervical and axillary lymph nodes metastasis is frequent.

4. Occurs most frequently in individuals above fourth decade, average age being fifty-six years.[98]

5. Malignant melanoma has male predilection, almost twice more common in men

Histologic features

Melanomas are characterized by the presence of atypical melanocytes at the basement membrane zone that tend to spread along the basal layer, proliferate upward throughout the epithelium and eventually invade the underlying connective tissue.[99] melanomas generally exhibit two growth phases: the radial growth phase and the vertical growth phase.

During the radial growth phase, malignant melanocytes spread laterally and superiorly, but remain confined within the epithelium. This is sometimes referred to as melanoma in situ. The vertical growth phase begins when the malignant cells invade the underlying connective tissue. In nodular melanomas, the radial growth phase is nonexistent or very short-lived.

Treatment

Oral melanomas usually have poor prognosis without any correlation with the depth of invasion, and most of them are ultimately fatal.[99] clinical staging helps in treatment planning.

Surgical excision is the only curative treatment, although protocols utilizing combination of treatment modalities like chemotherapy, radiotherapy, and immunotherapy may offer future alternative approaches for advanced lesions.

Sarcoma

Kaposi's sarcoma frequently occurs in the oral cavity of patients with acquired immunodeficiency syndrome (aids), particularly in the palate and the gingiva. Fibrosarcoma, lymphosarcoma and reticulum cell sarcoma of the gingiva are rare.[2]

Clinical features

1. The lesions start as small brown, purple or red macule that ultimately become nodular or Plaque-like. (Fig. 10).
2. Eventually the lesion gets ulcerated with bleeding which leads to interference with normal functions such as speaking, swallowing, and eating.

Pallavi Sharma, Dwiti Thanawala,
Alankrita Chaudhary, Himani Sharma

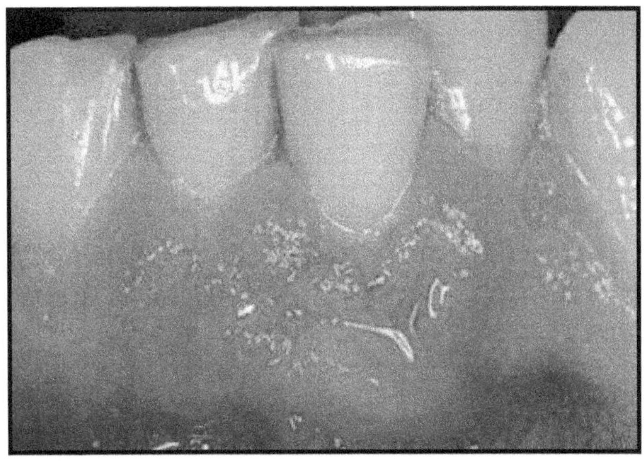

Fig. 10– Sarcoma of the gingiva

Histologic features

1. The histopathological features of early lesions are unremarkable, making it difficult to differentiate it from benign vascular lesion.

2. Well-established lesions demonstrate an interweaving spindle cell proliferation with small slit-like vascular spaces containing dispersed erythrocytes.

3. A characteristic but nonspecific feature is the presence of numerous hyaline globules or spheres, representing senescent erythrocytes[95]

Differential diagnosis

Individual lesions may be mistaken clinically as other vascular lesions such as hemangiomas or pyogenic granulomas.

Treatment

Oral lesions may be treated with intralesional chemotherapy or injection of sclerosing agents to control bleeding. [95]

Metastasis[2, 95]

It is uncommon for tumors to metastasize to the gingiva, with metastasis usually being noticed in the jawbones. Metastasis to oral soft tissues is present only in roughly 35% of cases.[95] on most occasions, metastasis occurs via blood-borne routes. Especially when the primary tumor is far from the oral cavity. When the primary site is located adjacent to oral structures metastasis may also occur via lymphatic channels.

The most common soft tissue sites for metastases in the oral cavity are the gingiva and tongue. Clinically, the soft tissue metastasis typically presents as a nodule or mass easily mistaken for a reactive lesion. In the gingiva, metastasis may involve the underlying alveolar leading to tooth mobility in adjoining regions, such as in tumors like adenocarcinoma of the colon, lung carcinoma, primary hepatocellular carcinoma, renal cell carcinoma, hypernephroma, chondrosarcoma and testicular tumor.

The resemblance of the microscopic appearance of the metastatic lesion with the primary lesion helps in conformation of the diagnosis. Patients with oral metastasis typically have a grave prognosis.

8. False Enlargement

False enlargements appear due to the growth in the size of the underlying dental or osseous tissues and aren't true enlargements of the gingival tissues. The gingiva typically shows no aberrant clinical features apart from the enormous growth in size. [2]

Underlying osseous lesions (Fig. 1)

Enlargement of the bone subjacent to the gingival area occurs most frequently in tori and exostoses, but it can also occur in fibrous dysplasia, paget's disease osteoma, osteosarcoma, cherubism, central giant cell granuloma and ameloblastoma. The gingiva can either look normal or may have inflammatory changes unrelated to the osseous lesions.

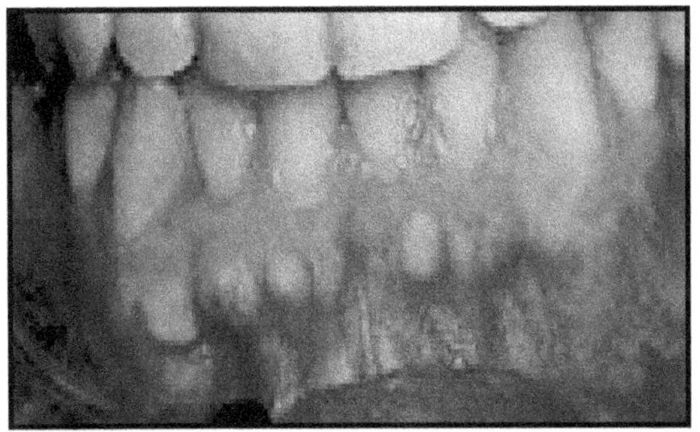

Fig 1–False gingival enlargement.

Developmental enlargement (Fig. 2)

During the various stages of eruption, especially in the primary dentition, the labial gingiva might show a bulbous marginal distortion which is caused because the bulk of the gingiva is superimposed on the prominence of the enamel in the apical half of the crown. This enlargement has been labelled developmental enlargement and frequently continues until the junctional epithelium has moved from the enamel to the cej. Developmental gingival enlargements are physiologic and typically cause no complications.

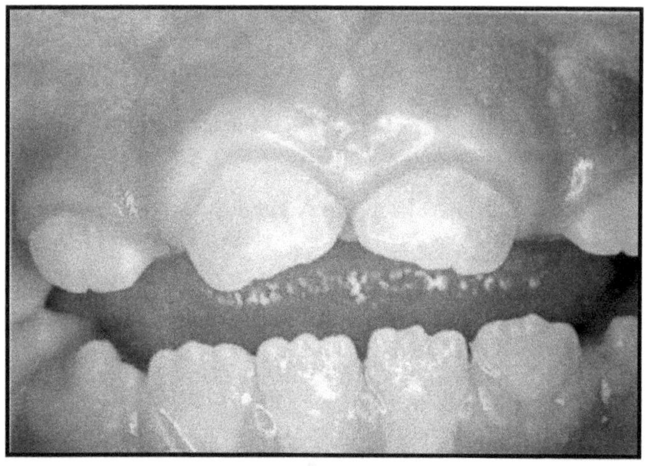

Fig. 2– Developmental gingival enlargement

However, if the development enlargement is complicated by marginal inflammation, it gives the impression of extensive gingival enlargement. Treatment to minimize the marginal inflammation is usually adequate in these cases.

Pallavi Sharma, Dwiti Thanawala,
Alankrita Chaudhary, Himani Sharma

9. Treatment Aspect

Bacterial plaque has been causally linked to various gingival and periodontal disease, thus the significance of appropriate oral hygiene instructions, assessment and reinforcement patient motivation, thorough oral hygiene practice at home, chlorhexidine mouthrinses and professional debridement has been emphasized. However, when the non-surgical method is ineffective, surgical elimination of the gingival overgrowth should be done (Fig. 1).

In certain cases, only reshaping of the gingiva by gingivoplasty would be adequate. Whereas in majority of cases, a more conclusive treatment is necessary, involving surgical removal of the excessive gingival tissue through either the gingivectomy procedure or flap surgery.

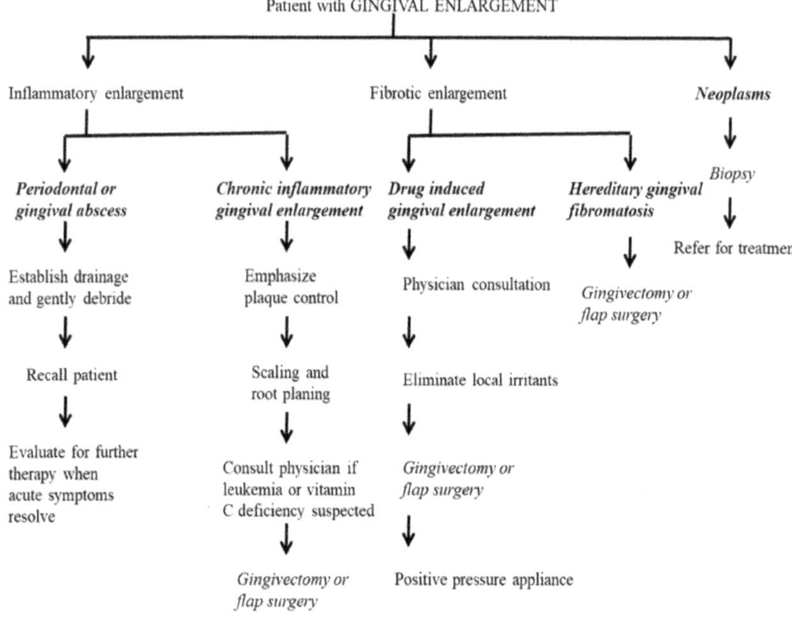

Fig. 1: Different treatment modalities for various gingival enlargements.

The clinician's decision to select between these surgical techniques is made after careful evaluation of various factors like the presence or absence of periodontitis and osseous defects, amount of keratinized gingiva, position of base of pockets with respect to the mucogingival junction, the amount of area requiring surgery (Fig. 2).

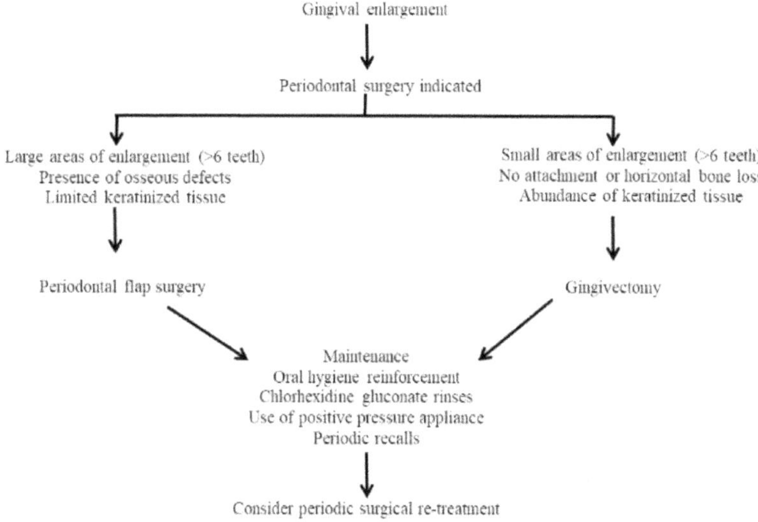

Fig. 2. Decision tree for surgical treatment of gingival enlargement

Gingivoplasty

Gingivoplasty is recontouring of the gingiva to produce physiologic gingival contours, with the objective of reshaping the gingiva in the absence of pockets. It may be performed surgically, or with electrocautery, rotary instruments or using lasers.[2]

Gingivectomy

Gingivectomy is the excisional elimination of the gingival tissue.[100] the gingivectomy procedure may be performed by scalpels, electrodes, chemicals or lasers.[2]

Surgical gingivectomy

I.   Pre-surgical phase[100]

Presurgical preparation is done to eliminate local factors and decrease the inflammatory component. The periodontal pockets are probed for depth and extent. Osseous topography is determined by bone sounding, as gingivectomy is contraindicated if osseous surgery is necessary. Adequate local anesthesia is required prior to the surgical procedure.

II.   Surgical phase

- Pocket marking[100]

A series of small bleeding points are made using a pocket marker to define the base of the pockets demarcating the pocket wall to be removed. Three points (mesial, middle, distal) are marked on both facial as well as lingual aspects (Fig. 3). The pocket marker is positioned into the pocket, parallel to the tooth. Once the base of the pocket is reached, the tissue is marked, and bleeding points are established forming the incision line. (Fig. 4).

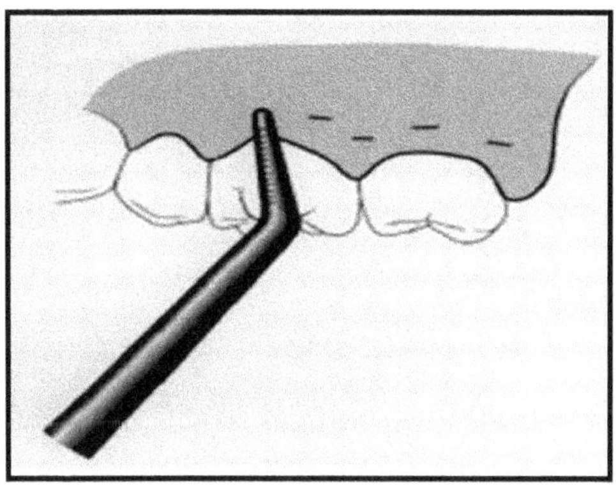

Fig 3– Pocket marker makes bleeding points that indicate pocket depth.

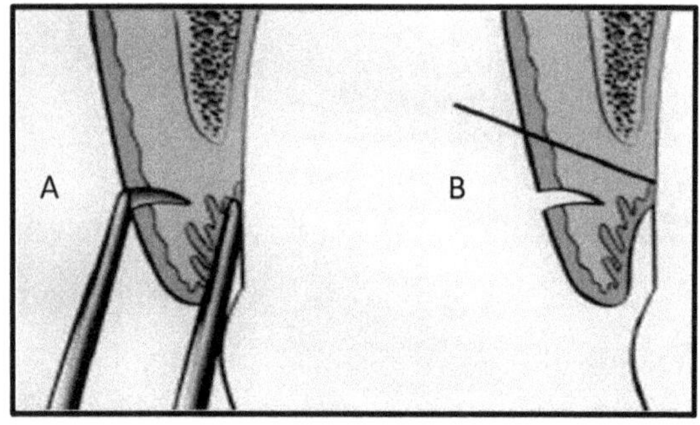

Fig 4

A) Pocket marker in position.

B) Beveled incision apical to the marking by

the pocket marker

Procedure 2 (Fig. 5 a-g)

1. Periodontal knives (e.g., kirkland knives) are utilized for incisions on the facial and lingual surfaces and those distal to the terminal tooth in the arch. Orban periodontal knives are used for supplemental interdental incisions, if necessary, and bard-parker knives #11 and 12 and scissors are used as auxiliary instruments.

2. The external bevel incision is initiated apical to the bleeding points, directed coronally to between the base of the pocket and the crest of the alveolar bone. The incision should be

placed as close as possible to the bone without exposing it to remove the soft tissue coronal to the bone.

3. The incision should be beveled at around 45° to the tooth surface to recreate the typical festooned pattern of the gingiva. Either continuous or discontinuous incisions may be employed.

4. The excised pocket wall is removed, and the area is thoroughly cleaned.

5. If granulation tissue is visible on the excised soft tissue, it is carefully curetted. Any remnant calculus and necrotic cementum is also removed to achieve a smooth and clean surface.

6. The surgical area is covered with a periodontal pack.

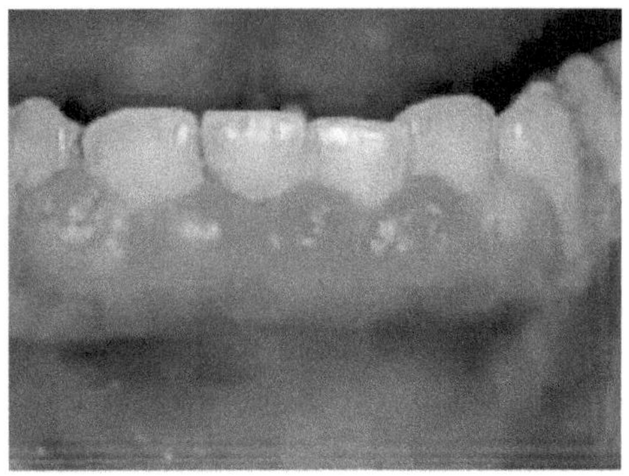

Fig. 5a – Pre-operative view showing enlarged gingival tissues.

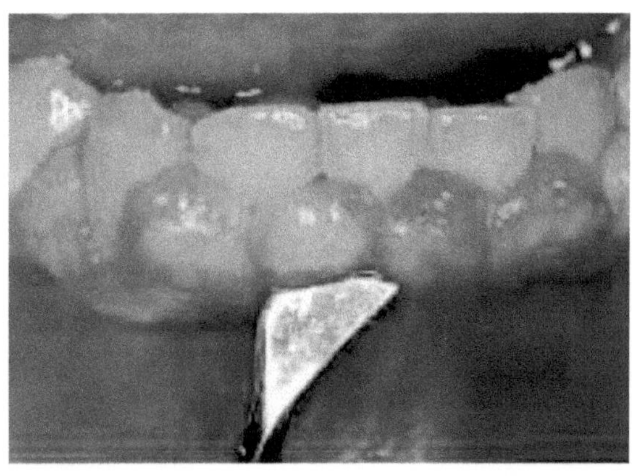

Fig. 5b – Internal bevel incision performed with a Kirkland knife.

Pallavi Sharma, Dwiti Thanawala,
Alankrita Chaudhary, Himani Sharma

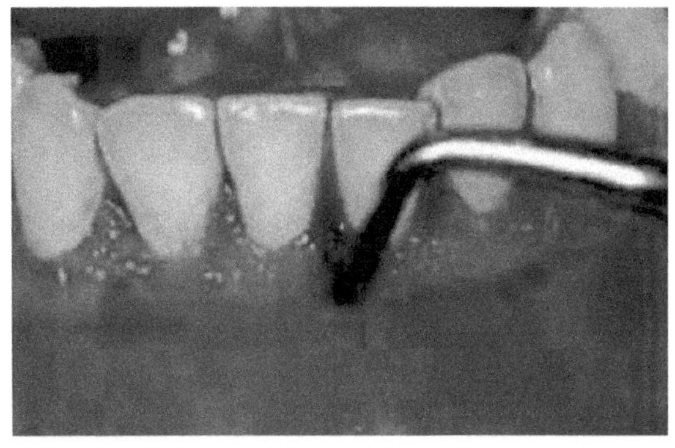

Fig. 5c –Supplemental interdental incisions with Orban's knife.

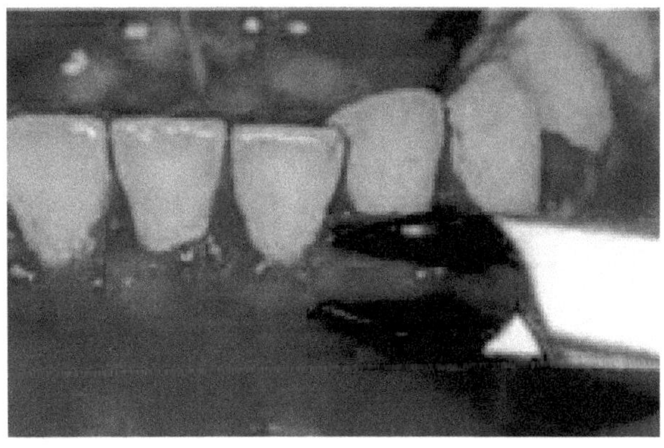

Fig. 5d – Gingivoplasty done with tissue nippers.

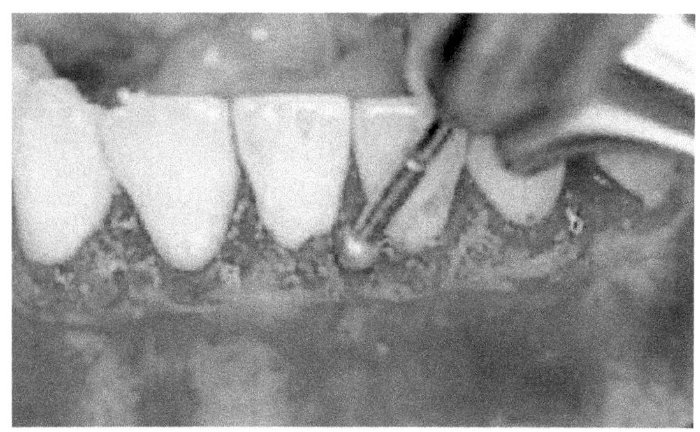

Fig. 5e Gingivoplasty done with round diamond
bur at high speed.

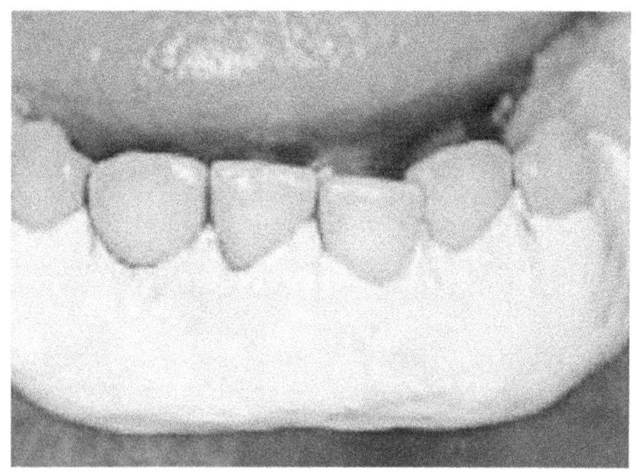

Fig. 5f – Placement of periodontal pack.

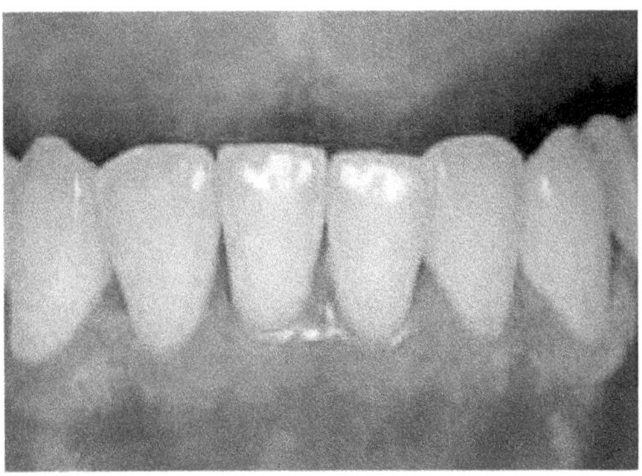

Fig. 5g– Surgical area 3 months post-operatively

Gingivectomy by electrosurgery

The excision of gingival enlargements and gingivoplasty is accomplished using needle electrodes along with diamond-shaped electrodes or small ovoid loop. A combined cutting and coagulating current are utilized. In all reshaping procedures, the activated electrode is moved in a concise shaving motion.

The ball electrode is used for hemostasis. Hemorrhage must be controlled by direct pressure first, thereafter the surface is lightly touched with a coagulating current. Electrosurgery is helpful for the control of isolated bleeding points. Bleeding points in the interproximal regions can be accessed using a thin, bar shaped electrode.

Advantages[2]

Electrosurgery facilitates adequate tissue contouring and controls hemorrhage.

Disadvantages[2]

1. Cannot be used in patients with poorly shielded or incompatible cardiac pacemakers.
2. It produces an unpleasant odor.
3. The heat generated by injudicious use may lead to tissue damage and loss of periodontal support. Irreversible damage to the alveolar bone may occur if the electrosurgery point touches the bone,
4. Areas of cementum burn are formed if the electrode touches the tooth root.

Therefore, the application of electrosurgery should be restricted to superficial procedures such as gingivoplasty, excision of gingival enlargements, and incision of periodontal abscesses.

Laser gingivectomy

The lasers most frequently used in dentistry are in the infrared range, the carbon dioxide (co2) with wavelengths of 10,600 nm and the neodymium: yttrium aluminum garnet (nd:yag), wavelengths of 1064 nm. They need to be combined with other visible lasers for the beam to be seen and targeted. The co2 laser beam has been employed for the excision of gingival enlargements; however, healing is delayed as compared with healing after conventional scalpel gingivectomy.[101]

The advantages of using laser gingivectomy over scalpel gingivectomy includes better coagulation leading to a dry surgical field and improved visualization, tissue surface sterilization and consequent decrease in bacteriemia, reduced edema and pain.

Studies concerning the co2 laser report mixed results for soft tissue healing when compared to scalpel gingivectomy. Some studies found a slower overall healing,[102] others found either slower initially but equal at two weeks, or equivalent to scalpel gingivectomy.[103] also, co2 laser-induced wounds in oral mucosa healed significantly faster than those created by Nd:YAG laser, but both heal slower than the conventional scalpel induced wounds.[102]

Gingivectomy by chemosurgery

The use of chemicals such as 5% paraformaldehyde or potassium hydroxide for removal of gingival growths are no longer in practice. The procedure had several disadvantages like inability to control the depth of action, inability to accomplish remodeling of the gingiva effectively, slower epithelialization and reformation of the junctional epithelium and reestablishment of the alveolar crest fiber system. [2]

The flap technique [2]

Flap technique sis the treatment of choice when of gingival enlargement occurs in larger areas (more than 6 teeth) or areas in the presence of osseous defects and loss of attachment.,

Procedure (Fig. 6)

1. Bone sounding of the underlying alveolar bone is done post local anesthesia, using a periodontal probe to establish the presence and extent of osseous defects.

2. The initial scalloped internal bevel incision is made using a #15 bard-parker blade, at least 3 mm coronal to the mucogingival junction, including the creation of new interdental papillae.

3. The same blade is used to thin the gingival tissues in a buccolingual direction to the mucogingival junction. When the blade establishes contact with the alveolar bone, a full-thickness or a partial-thickness flap is elevated.

4. The base of each papilla connecting the facial and the lingual incisions is incised, using an orban's knife.

5. The excised marginal and interdental tissue is removed with curettes. Tissue tags are removed, the tooth roots are thoroughly scaled and planed, and the bone is recontoured as required.

6. The flap is then sutured with an interrupted or a continuous mattress technique and the area is covered with periodontal dressing.

7. Sutures and periodontal dressing are removed after 1 week.

Chlorhexidine mouth rinses are advised to be used once or twice daily for 2 to 4 weeks. Meticulous home care, chlorhexidine mouth rinses, along with professional cleanings can reduce the pace and the extent of recurrence of gingival enlargement.

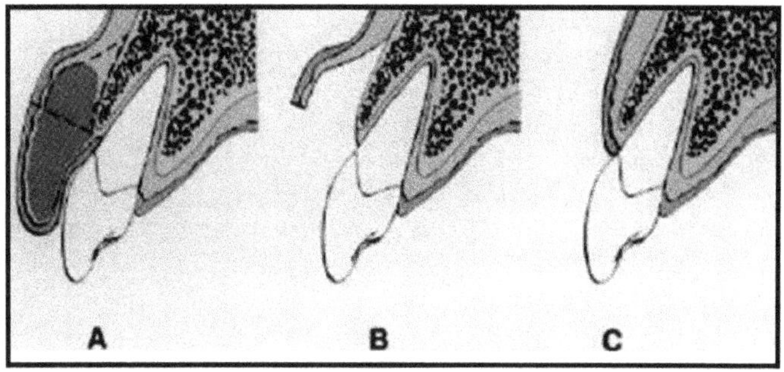

Fig. 6 – Diagram of periodontal flap surgery for gingival enlargement.

A) Initial reverse bevel incision followed by thinning of enlarged   gingival tissues; dotted lines represent incisions; shaded area represents tissue portion to be excised.

B) After flap elevation, enlarged portion of the gingival tissue is removed.

C) The flap is placed back and sutured.

10. Conclusion

Gingival enlargements are usually complex multifactorial in naturing occurring due to the several interactions between the host and the environment. Most of the gingival enlargements appear as an inflammatory response to bacterial plaque, however it is important to consider the role of systemic factors or conditions in increasing the patient's increased susceptibility to enlargement.

Gingival enlargements may lead to functional and esthetic impairment leading to significant decline in the patient's quality of life causing considerable emotional and social problems. Hence, a comprehensive and detailed history is necessary to rule out the existence of any hormonal imbalance, systemic disorders, drug history, hereditary pattern of occurrence etc.

Gingival enlargements have intense clinical, genetic, and biologic heterogeneity, as well as a wide array of etiologies exists for these conditions, hence extensive investigations might be necessary before achieving an appropriate diagnosis. This diagnostic design-up must follow a logical, stepwise approach. Prevention and management should be established on an understanding of the underlying etiopathogenesis, precise diagnosis, and appropriate risk management.

The multifarious etiology of gingival enlargements, large number of risk factors and risk indicators impacting the severity and extent of disease, makes the determination of pathogenesis difficult. Hence, newer molecular approaches are necessary to establish the pathogenesis of gingival enlargement and to provide necessary information for the design of future preventive and therapeutic modalities.[4]

11. References

1. Mariotti A. Dental Plaque-Induced Gingival Diseases. Ann Periodontol 1999; 4: 7-17.

2. Newman MG, Takei HH, Klokkevold PR, Carranza FA. Carranza's Clinical Periodontology, 10th edition. W. B. Saunders Company 2006.

3. Armitage GC. Development of a classification system for periodontal diseases and conditions. Ann Periodontol 1999; 4: 1.

4. Research, Science and Therapy Committee of the American Academy of Periodontology. Informational paper. Drug associated gingival enlargement. J Periodontol 2004; 75: 1424-1431.

5. Greenberg MS, Glick M. Burket's Oral medicine Diagnosis and Treatment, 10th edition. BC Decker 2003.

6. Meng HX. Periodontal abscess. Ann Periodontol 1999; 4, 79–83.

7. Herrera D, Rolda'n S, Sanz M: The periodontal abscess: A Review. J Clin Periodontol 2000; 27: 377–386.

8. DeWitt GV, Cobb CM & Killoy WJ. The acute periodontal abscess: microbial penetration of the tissue wall. Int J Periodontics Restorative Dent 1985; 1, 39–51.

9. Lindhe J, Lang NP, Karring T. Clinical Periodontology and Implant Dentistry, 5th edition. Blackwell Munksgaard.

10. Helovuo H, Hakkarainen K. & Paunio K. Changes in the prevalence of subgingival enteric rods, staphylococci and yeasts after treatment with penicillin and erythromycin. Oral Microbiol Immunol 1993; 8, 75–79.

11. Dello Russo MM The post-prophylaxis periodontal abscess: etiology and treatment. Int J Periodontics Restorative Dent 1985; 1, 29– 37.

12. Garrett S, Polson AM, Stoller NH, Drisko CL, Caton JG, Harrold CQ, Bogle G, Greenwell H, Lowenguth RA, Duke SP & DeRouen TA. Comparison of a bioabsorbable GTR barrier to a non-absorbable barrier in treating human class II furcation defects. A

multicenter parallel design randomized single blind study. J Periodontol 1997; 68, 667–675.

13. Gillette WB & Van House RL. Ill effects of improper oral hygiene procedures. J Am Dent Assoc 1980; 101: 476–481.

14. Newman MG & Sims TN. The predominant cultivable microbiota of the periodontal abscess. J Periodontol 1979; 50, 350–354.

15. Jaramillo A, Arce RM, Herrera D, Betancourth M, Botero JE, Contreras A. Clinical and microbiological characterization of periodontal abscesses. J Clin Periodontol 2005; 32: 1213–1218.

16. Ibbott CG, Kovach RJ & Carlson-Mann LD. Acute periodontal abscess associated with an immediate implant site in the maintenance phase. Int J Oral Maxillofac Implants 1993; 8: 699–702.

17. Hallmon WW, Rossmann JA. The role of drugs in pathogenesis of drug induced gingival overgrowth. A collective review of current concepts. Periodontol 2000 1999; 21: 176-196.

18. Lin Katia, Laura M. F. F. Guilhoto; Elza Márcia Targas Yacubian. Drug-induced gingival enlargement – Part II. Antiepileptic drugs: not only phenytoin is

involved.

J Epilepsy Clin Neurophysiol 2007; 13(2)

19. Seymour RA, Heasman PA, Mac Gregor IM. Drugs, diseases and periodontium, 1st edition. Oxford university press, 1992.

20. Tripathi KD. Essentials of Medical Pharmacology. Jaypee Brothers, 5th edition, 2003.

21. Seymour RA, Thoamson JM, Ellis JS. The pathogenesis of drug induced gingival overgrowth. J Clin Periodontol 1996; 23: 165-175.

22. Bredfeldt GW. Phenytoin-induced hyperplasia found in edentulous patients. J Am Dent Assoc 1992; 123: 61-64.

23. Hassell TM. Epilepsy and the oral manifestation of phenytoin therepy. New York: Karger 1981.

24. Kato T, Okahashi N, Kawai S, Kato T, Inaba H, Morisaki I, Amano A. Impaired degradation of matrix collagen in human gingival fibroblasts by antiepileptic drug phenytoin. J Periodontol 2005; 76: 941-950.

25. Modeer T, Mendez C, Dahllof G, Auduren I, Anderson G. Effect of phenytoin medication on the metabolism of epidermal growth factor receptor in

cultured gingival fibroblasts. J Periodontal Res 1990; 25: 120-127.

26. Dill RE, Miller K, Weil T, Lesley S, Farmer G, Iacopino A. Phenytoin increases gene expression for platelet-derived growth factor B chain in macrophages and monophages. J Periodontol 1993; 64: 169-173

27. Prasad VN, Chawla HS, Goyal A, Gauba K, Singhi P, Folic Acid and Phenytoin Induced Gingival Overgrowth - Is There A Preventive Effect. J Indian Soc Pedo Prev Dent 2004; 22(2): 82-91.

28. Katz J, Givol N, Chaushu G, Taicher S, Shemer J. Vigabatrin induced gingival overgrowth . J Clin Periodontol 1997; 24:180-182.

29. Seymour RA & Jacobs DJ. Cyclosporin and the gingival tissues. J Clin Periodontol 1992; 19: 1–11.

30. Marshall RI, Bartold PM. A clinical review of drug-induced gingival overgrowths. Australian Dental Journal 1999;44:(4):219-232

31. Rostock MH, Fry HR, Turner JE. Severe gingival overgrowth associated with cyclosporine therapy. J Periodontol 1986; 57: 294-299.

32. Thomason JM, Seymour RA & Rice N. The prevalence and severity of cyclosporin and nifedipine-

induced gingival overgrowth. J Clin Periodontol 1993; 20: 37–40.

33. Bokenkamp A, Bohnhorst B, Beier C, Albers N, Offner G & Brodehl J. Nifedipine aggravates cyclosporine A-induced gingival hyperplasia. Pediatric Nephrology 1994; 8: 181–185.

34. Margiotta V, Pizzo I, Pizzo G, & Barbaro A. Cyclosporin and nifedipine-induced gingival overgrowth in renal transplant patients: correlations with periodontal and pharmacological parameters, and HLA-antigens. J Oral Pathol Med 1996; 25: 128–134.

35. Wondimu B, Sandberg J & Modeer T. Gingival overgrowth in renal transplant patients administered cyclosporin A in mixture or in capsule form. A longitudinal study. Clin Transplant 1996; 10: 71– 76.

36. Pernu, EH, Knuuttila MLE, Huttenen KRH & Tiilikainen ASK. Drug-induced gingival overgrowth and class II major histocompatibility antigens. Transplantation 1994; 57: 1811–1813.

37. Das SJ, Parkar M, Olsen I. Upregulation of keratinocyte growth factor in cyclosporin A induced gingival overgrowth. J Periodontol 2001; 72: 745-752.

38. Gnoatto N, Lotufo RFM, Toffoletto O, Marquezini M. Gene expression of extracellular matrix proteoglycans

in human cyclosporin induced gingival overgrowth J Periodontol 2003; 74: 1747-1753.

39. Myrillas T, Linden G, Marley J, Irwin C. Cyclosporin A regulates interleukin 1 β and interleukin 6 expression in gingiva: implications for gingival overgrowth. J Periodontol 1999; 70: 294-300

40. Chin YT, Chen YT, Tu HP, Shen EC, Chiang CY, Gau CH, Nieh S, Fu E. Upregulation of expression of epidermal growth factor and its receptor in gingiva upon cyclosporin A treatment. J Periodontol 2006; 77: 647-656.

41. Boltchi FE, Rees T, Iacopino A. Cyclosporin A-induced gingival overgrowth: A comprehensive review. Quintessence Int 1999; 30: 775-783.

42. Daley TD, Wysocki GP & Day C Clinical and pharmacologic correlations in cyclosporine-induced gingival hyperplasia. Oral Surg Oral Med Oral Pathol Oral Radiol Endod 1986; 62: 417–421

43. Barclay S, Thomason JM, Idle JR, Seymour RA. The incidence and severity of nifedipine induced gingival overgrowth. J Clin Periodontol 1992; 19: 311-314.

44. Seymour RA. Calcium channel blockers and gingival overgrowth. Br Dent J 1991; 170: 376-379.

45. Seymour RA, Ellis JS, Thomason JM, Monkman S & Idle JR. Amlodipine- induced gingival overgrowth. J Clin Periodontol 1994; 21: 281–283.

46. Desai P, Silver JG. Drug induced gingival enlargements. J Canad Dent Assn 1998; 64(4): 263-267

47. Miller C, Damm D. Incidence of verapamil induced gingival hyperplasia in a dental population. J Periodontol 1992; 63: 453-546

48. Valsecchi R, Cainelli T. Gingival hyperplasia induced by erythromycin. Acta Derm Venereol 1992; 72: 157.

49. Seymour RA, Ellis JS, Thomason JM. Risk factors for drug-induced gingival overgrowth. J Clin Periodontol 2000; 27: 217–223.

50. Thomason JM, Ellis JS, Kelly PJ & Seymour RA. Nifedipine pharmacological variables as risk factors for gingival overgrowth in organ-transplant patients. Clin Oral Investig 1997; 1: 35– 39.

51. Sooriyamoorthy M, Gower DB & Eley BM. Androgen metabolism in gingival hyperplasia induced by nifedipine and cyclosporin. J Periodont Res 1990; 25, 25–30.

52. Ellis J, Seymour R, Steele J, Robertson P & Butler T. Prevalence of gingival overgrowth induced by calcium

channel blockers: a community based study. J Periodontol 1999; 70: 63–67.

53. Hassell TM & Hefti AF. Drug induced gingival overgrowth: old problem, new problem. Crit Rev Oral Biol M 1991; 2: 103–137.

54. Ball DE, McLaughlin WS, Seymour RA & Kamali F. Plasma and saliva concentrations of phenytoin and 5-(4-hydroxyphenyl)- 5-phenylhydantoin in relation to the incidence and severity of phenytoin-induced gingival overgrowth in epileptic patients. J Periodontol 1996; 67: 597–602.

55. Niimi A, Tohnai I, Kaneda T, Takouchi M & Nagura H. Immunohistochemical analysis of effects of cyclosporine A on gingival epithelium. J Oral Pathol Med 1990; 19: 397–403.

56. McLaughlin WS, Ball DE, Seymour RA, Kamali F & White K. The pharmacokinetics of phenytoin in gingival crevicular fluid and plasma in relation to gingival overgrowth. J Clin Periodontol 1995; 22: 942–945.

57. Pernu HE, Pernu LM & Knuuttila ML. Effect of periodontal treatment on gingival overgrowth among cyclosporine A-treated renal transplant recipients. J Periodontol 1993; 64: 1098–1100.

58. Hassell TM & Page RC. The major metabolite of phenytoin (Dilantin) induces gingival overgrowth in cats. J Periodont Res 1978; 13: 280– 282.

59. Varga E, Lennon MA & Mair LH. Pre-transplant gingival hyperplasia predicts severe cyclosporin-induced gingival overgrowth in renal transplant patients. J Clin Periodontol 1998; 25: 225–230.

60. Ingles E, Rossmann JA, Caffesse R. New clinical index for drug induced gingival overgrowth. Quintessence Int 1999; 30: 467-473

61. Ellis JS, Seymour RA, Robertson P, Butler TJ, Thomason JM. Photographic scoring of gingival overgrowth. J Clin Periodontol 2001; 28: 81-85

62. Mavrogiannis M, Ellis JS, Thomason JM, Seymour RA. The management of drug induced gingival overgrowth. J Clin Periodontol 2006; 33: 434–439.

63. Camargo PM, Melnick PR, Pirih FQM, Lagos R & Takei H. Treatment of drug induced gingival enlargement: aesthetic and functional considerations Periodontol 2000 2001; 27: 131–138.

64. Linares LP, Marqués NA, Aytés LB, Escoda CG. Effectiveness of substituting cyclosporin A with tacrolimus in reducing gingival overgrowth in renal

transplant patients. Med Oral Patol Oral Cir Bucal. 2009;14 (9): e429-33.

65. Spolidorio LC, Holzhausen M, Spolidorio DM, Nassar C, Nassar P, Muscara MN. Cyclosporine but not tacrolimus significantly increases salivary cytokine contents in rats J Periodontol 2005; 76: 1520-1525.

66. Mascarenhas P, Gapski R, Al-Shammari K, Wang H-L. Influence of sex hormones on the periodontium. J Clin Periodontol 2003; 30: 671–681.

67. Mariotti A. Sex steroid hormones and cell dynamics in the periodontium. Crit Rev Oral Biol M 1994; 5(1): 27-53

68. Rose LF, Genco RJ, Maeley BL, Cohen DW. Periodontal Medicine. BC Decker Inc 2000

69. Gusberti FA, Mombelli A, Lang NE Minder CE. Changes in subgingival microbiota during puberty. J Clin Periodontal 1990; 17: 685-692.

70. Kornman KS, Loesche WJ. The subgingival flora during pregnancy. J Periodontol 1980; 15: 111-122.

71. Raber-Durlacher JE, Leene W, Palmer-Bouva CCR. Experimental gingivitis during pregnancy and post partum: immunohistochemical aspects. J Periodontol 1993; 64: 211-218.

72. Kinnby B, Matsson L, Astedt B. Aggravation of gingival inflammatory symptoms during pregnancy associated with the concentration of activator inhibitor type 2 (PAI-2) in gingival fluid. J Periodontal Res 1996; 31(4): 271-277.

73. Bhashkar SN, Jacoway JR. Pyogenic granuloma. Clinical features, incidence, histology, and results of treatment. Report of 242 cases. J Oral Surg1966; 24: 39 1-8.

74. Oeffinger KC. Scurvy: more than historical relevance. American Family Physician 1993; 48, 609–613.

75. Shafer WG, Hine MK, Levy BM. A Textbook of Oral Pathology, 4th edition. Saunders 2000.

76. Woolfe SN, Hume WR. & Kenney, EB. Ascorbic acid and periodontal disease: a review of the literature. The Journal of the Western Society of Periodontology/Periodontal Abstracts 1980; 28: 44–56.

77. Serio FG, Siegel MA, Slade BE. Plasma cell gingivitis of unusual origin-A case report. J Periodontol 1991; 62(6):390-393.

78. Sukumaran A. Plasma Cell Gingivitis Among Herbal Toothpaste Users: A Report of Three Cases. J Contemp Dent Pract 2007; 8 (4): 60-66.

79. Nitta H, Kameyama Y, Ishikawa 1: Unusual gingival enlargement with rapidly progressive periodontitis. Report of a case. J Periodontol 1993; 64:1008.

80. Patil K, Mahima VG, Lahari K . Extraginigval pyogenic granuloma - A Case Report. Indian J Dent Res 2006; 17: 199-202.

81. Wu J, Fantasia JE, Kaplan R. Oral manifestations of acute myelomonocytic leukemia: A case report and review of classification of leukemia. J Periodontal 2002; 73: 664-668.

82. Serhat Demirer, Hakan Özdemir, Mehmet Şencan, and Ismail Marakoglu, Gingival Hyperplasia as an Early Diagnostic Oral Manifestation in Acute Monocytic Leukemia: A Case Report. Eur J Dent. 2007; 1(2): 111–114.

83. Stafford R, Sonis S, Lockhart P, Sonis A. Oral Pathoses as diagnostic indicators in leukemia. Oral Surg Oral Med Oral Pathol 1980; 50: 134-139.

84. Neville BW, Damm DD, Allen CM, Bouquot JE. Oral and Maxillofacial pathology, 2nd edition. WB Saunders company 2002.

85. Hernandez G, Serrano C, Porras L, Lopez-Pintor R, Rubio L, and Yanes J. Strawberry-Like Gingival

Tumor as the First Clinical Sign of Wegener's Granulomatosis. J Periodontol 2008; 79:1297-1303.

86. Patten SF, Tomecki KJ. Wegener's granulomatosis: Cutaneous and oral mucosal disease. J Am Acad Dermatol 1993; 28: 710-718.

87. Coletta RD, Graner E. Hereditary systemic fibromatosis: A Systematic Review. J Periodontol 2006; 77: 753-764.

88. Hart TC, Zhang Y, Gorry MC. A mutation in the SOS1 gene causes hereditary gingival fibromatosis type 1. Am J Hum Genet 2002; 70: 943-954.

89. Tipton DA, Howell KJ, Dabbous MK. Increased proliferation, collagen, and fibronectin production by hereditary gingival fibromatosis fibroblasts. J Periodontol 1997; 68: 524-530.

90. Martelli-Junior H, Cotrim P, Graner E, Sauk JJ, Coletta RD. Effect of transforming growth factorbeta1, interleukin-6, and interferon-gamma on the expression of type I collagen, heat shock protein 47, matrix metalloproteinase (MMP)-1 and MMP-2 by fibroblasts from normal gingiva and hereditary gingival fibromatosis. J Periodontol 2003; 74: 296-306.

91. McCarthy FP. A clinical and pathological study of oral disease. JAMA 1941; 16: 116

92. Bernick S. Growth of the gingiva and palate. II. Connective tissue tumors. Oral Surg 1948; 1:1098.

93. Bhaskar SN, Levin MP. Histopathology of the human gingiva (study based on 1269 biopsies). J Periodontol 1973; 44:3-17.

94. Abitbol TE, Santi E. Peripheral ossifying fibroma – Literature update and clinical case. Periodontal Clin Investig 1997; 19: 36-37.

95. Fowler CB. Benign and malignant neoplasms of the periodontium. Periodontol 2000 1999; 21: 33.

96. Garewal HS, Meyskens FL Jr, Killen D, Reeves D, Kiersch TA, Elletson H, Strosberg A, King D, Steinbronn K. Response of oral leukoplakia to beta-carotene. J Clin Oncol 1990; 8: 1715-1720

97. Heller AN, Klein A, Barocas A. Squamous cell carcinoma of the gingiva presenting as an endoperiodontic lesion. J Periodontol 1991; 62: 573-575.

98. Barker BF, Carpenter WM, Daniels TE, Kahn MA, Leider AS, Lozada-Nur E Lynch DP, Melrose R, Merrell P, Morton T, Peters E, Regezi JA, Richards SD, Rick GM, Rohrer MD, Slater L, Stewart JC, Tomich CE, Vickers RA, Wood NK, Young SK. Oral

mucosal melanomas. Oral Surg Oral Med Oral Pathol Oral Radiol Endod 1997: 83; 672-679.

99. Umeda M, Shimada K. Primary malignant melanoma of the oral cavity - its histological classification and treatment. Br J Oral Maxillofac Surg 1994: 32: 39-47.

100. Cohen ES. Atlas of cosmetic and Reconstructive periodontal surgery, 3rd edition. BC Decker Inc 2007.

101. Research, Science and Therapy Committee of the American Academy of Periodontology. Lasers in Periodontics. J Periodontol 2002; 73:1231- 1239.

102. Lippert BM, Teymoortash A, Folz BJ, Werner JA. Wound healing after laser treatment of oral and oropharyngeal cancer. Lasers Med Sci 2003;18: 36-42.

103. Arashiro DS, Rapley JW, Cobb CM, Killoy WJ. Histologic evaluation of porcine skin incisions produced by CO2 laser, electrosurgery and scalpel. Int J Periodontics Restorative Dent 1996; 16: 479-491.